# STRATEGIC APPROACH TO EVALUATION OF PROGRAMS IMPLEMENTED UNDER THE TOM LANTOS AND HENRY J. HYDE U.S. GLOBAL LEADERSHIP AGAINST HIV/AIDS, TUBERCULOSIS, AND MALARIA REAUTHORIZATION ACT OF 2008

Committee on Planning the Assessment/Evaluation of Programs Implemented
Under the U.S. Global Leadership Against HIV/AIDS, Tuberculosis,
and Malaria Reauthorization Act of 2008

Board on Global Health
Board on Children, Youth, and Families

INSTITUTE OF MEDICINE *AND*
NATIONAL RESEARCH COUNCIL
*OF THE NATIONAL ACADEMIES*

THE NATIONAL ACADEMIES PRESS
Washington, D.C.
**www.nap.edu**

**THE NATIONAL ACADEMIES PRESS    500 Fifth Street, N.W.    Washington, DC 20001**

NOTICE: The project that is the subject of this report was approved by the Governing Board of the National Research Council, whose members are drawn from the councils of the National Academy of Sciences, the National Academy of Engineering, and the Institute of Medicine. The members of the committee responsible for the report were chosen for their special competences and with regard for appropriate balance.

This study was supported by Contract No. SAQMMA09M0693 (STAT-3977) between the National Academy of Sciences and Department of State. Any opinions, findings, conclusions, or recommendations expressed in this publication are those of the author(s) and do not necessarily reflect the view of the organizations or agencies that provided support for this project.

International Standard Book Number-13: 978-0-309-15393-5
International Standard Book Number-10: 0-309-15393-X

Additional copies of this report are available from the National Academies Press, 500 Fifth Street, N.W., Lockbox 285, Washington, DC 20055; (800) 624-6242 or (202) 334-3313 (in the Washington metropolitan area); Internet, http://www.nap.edu.

For more information about the Institute of Medicine, visit the IOM home page at: **www.iom.edu.**

Suggested citation: IOM and NRC (Institute of Medicine and National Research Council). 2010. *Strategic approach to the evaluation of programs implemented under the Tom Lantos and Henry J. Hyde U.S. Global Leadership Against HIV/AIDS, Tuberculosis, and Malaria Reauthorization Act of 2008.* Washington, DC: The National Academies Press.

# THE NATIONAL ACADEMIES
*Advisers to the Nation on Science, Engineering, and Medicine*

The **National Academy of Sciences** is a private, nonprofit, self-perpetuating society of distinguished scholars engaged in scientific and engineering research, dedicated to the furtherance of science and technology and to their use for the general welfare. Upon the authority of the charter granted to it by the Congress in 1863, the Academy has a mandate that requires it to advise the federal government on scientific and technical matters. Dr. Ralph J. Cicerone is president of the National Academy of Sciences.

The **National Academy of Engineering** was established in 1964, under the charter of the National Academy of Sciences, as a parallel organization of outstanding engineers. It is autonomous in its administration and in the selection of its members, sharing with the National Academy of Sciences the responsibility for advising the federal government. The National Academy of Engineering also sponsors engineering programs aimed at meeting national needs, encourages education and research, and recognizes the superior achievements of engineers. Dr. Charles M. Vest is president of the National Academy of Engineering.

The **Institute of Medicine** was established in 1970 by the National Academy of Sciences to secure the services of eminent members of appropriate professions in the examination of policy matters pertaining to the health of the public. The Institute acts under the responsibility given to the National Academy of Sciences by its congressional charter to be an adviser to the federal government and, upon its own initiative, to identify issues of medical care, research, and education. Dr. Harvey V. Fineberg is president of the Institute of Medicine.

The **National Research Council** was organized by the National Academy of Sciences in 1916 to associate the broad community of science and technology with the Academy's purposes of furthering knowledge and advising the federal government. Functioning in accordance with general policies determined by the Academy, the Council has become the principal operating agency of both the National Academy of Sciences and the National Academy of Engineering in providing services to the government, the public, and the scientific and engineering communities. The Council is administered jointly by both Academies and the Institute of Medicine. Dr. Ralph J. Cicerone and Dr. Charles M. Vest are chair and vice chair, respectively, of the National Research Council.

www.national-academies.org

# Reviewers

This report has been reviewed in draft form by individuals chosen for their diverse perspectives and technical expertise, in accordance with procedures approved by the National Research Council's Report Review Committee. The purpose of this independent review is to provide candid and critical comments that will assist the institution in making its published report as sound as possible and to ensure that the report meets institutional standards for objectivity, evidence, and responsiveness to the study charge. The review comments and draft manuscript remain confidential to protect the integrity of the deliberative process. We wish to thank the following individuals for their review of this report:

**Stefano Bertozzi,** Bill & Melinda Gates Foundation
**Greg Bisson,** University of Pennsylvania School of Medicine
**Thomas Coates,** University of California Los Angeles, School of Medicine
**Lola Dare,** CHESTRAD International
**Victor DeGruttola,** Harvard School of Public Health
**Theresa Díaz Vargas,** United Nations Children's Fund
**Johanna Dwyer,** Tufts University School of Medicine and Friedman School of Nutrition Science & Policy
**Robert Hecht,** Results for Development Institute
**Phyllis Kanki,** Harvard School of Public Health
**Kathy Marconi,** University of Maryland University College
**Peter Mugyenyi,** Joint Clinical Research Center, Kampala, Uganda
**Robert R. Redfield,** University of Maryland School of Medicine

Although the reviewers listed above have provided many constructive comments and suggestions, they were not asked to endorse the conclusions or recommendations nor did they see the final draft of the report before its release. The review of this report was overseen by **Bernard Guyer,** Johns Hopkins University Bloomberg School of Public Health and **Edward Perrin,** Emeritus, University of Washington. Appointed by the National Research Council and Institute of Medicine, they were responsible for making certain that an independent examination of this report was carried out in accordance with institutional procedures and that all review comments were carefully considered. Responsibility for the final content of this report rests entirely with the authoring committee and the institution.

# Acknowledgments

The committee would like to acknowledge the diverse and important contributions of the many individuals whose assistance is reflected in this report. First, the Committee would like to thank the Office of the U.S. Global AIDS Coordinator and the congressional staff who provided information, guidance, and support. The committee also greatly benefited from the time and expertise of those who met with committee delegations and participated in public information-gathering sessions. These individuals are listed in full in Appendix C.

There are a number of individuals who were critical for the administrative and logistical success of this project. For help with scheduling and communication, the committee would like to thank Mary Rybczynski, Rachel White, Lola Adedokun, Nancy Leonard, Polina Royzman-Tabak, Fortuna Salinas, Tanya Davis-Powell, Cindy Ogasawara, Elvira Bustamante, Audrey Palix, Aubrey Celeste C. Musngi-Anouar, Cindy Chu, and Sharon Abbruscato. The committee is also grateful to Anthony Mavrogiannis and the staff at Kentlands travel for their assistance with the travel needs of this project. The committee would also like to thank Kristin Shaw and Megan Perez for their excellent work on this project as interns at the Institute of Medicine. Carmen Mundaca also deserves special mention for her valuable research and analytic contributions during the time she devoted to the project as an intern within her doctoral training program.

# Preface

By the first decade of the 21st century, the world had been grappling with the HIV/AIDS pandemic for nearly three decades. The countries hardest hit in terms of morbidity and mortality remain in sub-Saharan Africa, home to an estimated two-thirds of people living with HIV infection. Although international aid has increased substantially since the beginning of the pandemic and national government expenditure for HIV prevention, treatment, care, and capacity building activities also increased in the most affected countries, there remains a funding gap relative to the estimated need.

In 2003, Congress mandated a study to be conducted by the Institute of Medicine (IOM) to assess the progress of the implementation of the programs and aid offered in a major new U.S initiative that became known as the President's Emergency Plan for AIDS Relief (PEPFAR). The findings and recommendations of that study informed the processes, policies, and activities of the program and the reauthorization legislation,[1] known in short as the Lantos–Hyde Act of 2008. This reauthorized legislation mandated another study by the IOM to assess the performance of United States-assisted global HIV/AIDS programs and evaluate the impact on health of prevention, treatment, and care efforts that are supported by United States funding (for a complete description of the elements to be considered in the assessment and evaluation, see the Statement of Task in Appendix A). In addition to informing Congress and the Department of State, this newly-mandated, evidence-based IOM study will provide the scientific community, program implementers, policy makers, civil society, people living with and affected by HIV/AIDS, and international stakeholders in global public health with a rigorous, non-partisan, multidisciplinary, and independent evaluation of the PEPFAR program.

This report outlines the design plan for the evaluation of this evolving program that has geographically expanded to more than twice the number of countries funded at the time of the first evaluation. This new evaluation is complicated by not only its scale, but also the diversity created by the characteristics and complexities of each country in which the program operates. The dynamism as a program in operation parallel to the evaluation itself—and the challenges that presents—also add complexity. The context in which PEPFAR operates has also shifted, with a more recent emphasis on transitioning from an emergency response to a longer-term model of sustainability, promoting country ownership, and strengthening health systems. PEPFAR also has a new place within the context of international funding as part of the new U.S. Global Health Initiative (GHI). Less than a year after PEPFAR was reauthorized, the Obama Administration launched the GHI—a new 6-year (2009–2014), $63 billion government-wide effort to develop a comprehensive U.S. global health strategy (these funds include PEPFAR funds). The GHI includes and builds on the success of PEPFAR, but also includes other global health challenges in a more coordinated approach. As such, the GHI is expected to affect the way in which all U.S. global health programs operate, including PEPFAR.

This plan includes an illustration of the types of questions that could be addressed in the evaluation, partitioning and elaborating the areas of interest described in the statement of task.

---

[1] Tom Lantos and Henry J. Hyde United States Global Leadership Against HIV/AIDS, Tuberculosis, and Malaria Reauthorization Act of 2008, Public Law 110-293, 110th Cong., 2nd sess. (July 30, 2008).

The ability to answer these evaluation questions will depend on the availability of timely and quality data from the Department of State's Office of the Global AIDS Coordinator and other sources such as other federal agencies, U.S. Country Teams and implementing partners, other donors, and other international stakeholders including the Global Fund to Fight AIDS, Tuberculosis, and Malaria, the World Health Organization, the Joint United Nations Programme on HIV/AIDS, and the United Nations Children's Fund. While the evaluation questions illustrated in this plan will undergo further refinement and prioritization, they are presented here to facilitate an understanding of not only the type of data needed from the numerous sources, but also the processes and temporal complexities inherent in responding to the committee's charge.

The evaluation will be conducted between 2010 and 2012, with a report of the committee's findings and recommendations issued in 2012. It will provide insights into the contributions of the investment made by the United States through PEPFAR to improve and save lives of men, women, adolescents, and children living with and affected by HIV/AIDS in developing countries.

In the current time of global economic recessions, limited resources, and stated intentions to transition to a more sustainable and country-owned response to the pandemic, an even more urgent priority must be accorded to the identification, dissemination, and scale-up of the most effective strategies for preventing new HIV infections and meeting the myriad needs of people already living with HIV/AIDS. The committee hopes to contribute to this knowledge and understanding.

The committee extends its gratitude to all those who provided information to assist in the planning committee's work. In our initial data gathering, we have been able to forge positive relationships with major global stakeholders. Perhaps the most important milestone in this planning phase is the commitment of those major global stakeholders to share their data, analyses, and other invaluable information with the IOM, thereby modeling indispensable international collaboration to collectively address and understand critical issues and outcomes related to the pandemic.

In closing, I would like to express my appreciation to the study staff for their superb work on this project and to the members of the committee for the time and energy they gave so generously to this project, for the expertise they contributed, and for their participation in robust discourse and deliberation.

> Robert E. Black, *Chair*
> Committee on Planning the Assessment/Evaluation
>   of HIV/AIDS Programs Implemented Under the
>   U.S. Global Leadership Against HIV/AIDS,
>   Tuberculosis, and Malaria Reauthorization Act of
>   2008

# Contents

# Tables, Figures, and Boxes

## TABLES

## FIGURES

## BOXES

# Acronyms and Abbreviations

| | |
|---|---|
| AEI | African Education Initiative |
| AIDS | acquired immune deficiency syndrome |
| APR | annual program results |
| ART | antiretroviral therapy |
| ARV | antiretroviral |
| BCC | behavior change communication |
| CD4 | cluster of differentiation 4 |
| CDC | U.S. Centers for Disease Control and Prevention |
| COP | country operational plan |
| COPRS | Country Operational Plan Reporting System |
| CRC | Committee on the Rights of the Child |
| CSW | commercial sex worker |
| CTX | cotrimoxazole |
| DHS | Demographic and Health Surveys |
| DoS | U.S. Department of State |
| EID | early infant diagnosis of HIV |
| FY | fiscal year |
| GHI | The U.S. Global Health Initiative |
| Global Fund | The Global Fund to Fight AIDS, Tuberculosis, and Malaria |
| HAPSAT | HIV/AIDS Program Sustainability Analysis Tool |
| HIV | human immunodeficiency virus |
| IDU | injecting drug user |
| IOM | U.S. Institute of Medicine |
| IPTp | intermittent preventive treatment of malaria for pregnant women |
| ITNs | insecticide-treated nets |
| M&E | monitoring and evaluation |
| MDG | Millennium Development Goal |
| MICS | Multiple Indicator Cluster Survey |
| MSM | men who have sex with men |
| NGO | non-governmental organization |
| OECD | Organisation for Economic Co-operation and Development |
| OGAC | Office of the U.S. Global AIDS Coordinator |
| OI | opportunistic infection |
| OMB | Office of Management and Budget |
| PCR | polymerase chain reaction |
| PEP | post-exposure prophylaxis |
| PEPFAR | The President's Emergency Plan for AIDS Relief |
| PEPFAR I | The President's Emergency Plan for AIDS Relief (2004–2008) |
| PEPFAR II | The President's Emergency Plan for AIDS Relief (2009–2013) |
| PHE | public health evaluation |
| PLWHA | people living with HIV/AIDS |
| PMI | The President's Malaria Initiative |

| PMTCT | prevention of mother-to-child transmission |
| PrEP | pre-exposure prophylaxis |
| SI | strategic information |
| SPRs | semi-annual progress results |
| TAB | Technical Advisory Board |
| TB | tuberculosis |
| TWG | Technical Working Group |
| UNAIDS | United Nations Joint Programme on HIV/AIDS |
| UNGASS | United Nations General Assembly Special Session |
| UNICEF | United Nations Children's Fund |
| USAID | United States Agency for International Development |
| USG | United States Government |
| WHO | World Health Organization |

# Summary of Key Messages

Since 2003, the United States has supported programs to combat global HIV/AIDS through an initiative that is known as the President's Emergency Plan for AIDS Relief (PEPFAR). The Lantos–Hyde Reauthorization Act of 2008 mandated a study by the Institute of Medicine (IOM) to assess and evaluate the performance and progress of the PEPFAR program and the impact on health of the program's activities, and to make recommendations to improve the U.S. government response to global HIV/AIDS.

As the first phase of this study, the IOM was charged to form an ad hoc committee to develop a plan for the evaluation and to issue a short report to the U.S. Congress on the plan's proposed design, taking into consideration the requirements for the congressionally mandated study (stated in Appendix A). This report presents an overview of the strategic approach and conceptual framework for the assessment and evaluation of PEPFAR. A transition period for operational planning will take place during congressional review of the strategic approach described in this report. In this operational planning phase, IOM staff, planning committee members, and consultants will carry out activities to further develop and refine the plan and to inform and prepare for the implementation of the evaluation. The evaluation itself will be conducted beginning in the fall of 2010, with a report of the findings and recommendations to be issued in 2012. The IOM will convene a new ad-hoc committee, with significant overlap from the membership of the planning committee, to conduct the evaluation as a consensus study.

The following key messages summarize the major elements of the evaluation approach.

- A program impact pathway reflects the rationale for how PEPFAR inputs and activities, including services, capacity building, technical assistance, and policy development, can be plausibly linked to effects on HIV-specific health impacts.
  - The program impact pathway contains five major elements: investments or **inputs** to the program; **activities** that provide services and support to those in need; **outputs** from these activities; **outcomes** that are measurable intermediate effects; and the ultimate goal of health **impact**.
  - This approach supports an assessment of whether the program is performing in the way it is intended along the full range of its implementation, rather than simply an evaluation of its ultimate impact. This will allow for refined conclusions about elements of the program that are functioning well or that could be improved to result in a greater impact on health.

- Within countries that receive PEPFAR support, a wide range of factors affect the implementation of the program and health outcomes, including cultural, societal, geographical, and political factors and influences, as well as the presence of investments and activities from a range of other external and country-level sources that are aimed at achieving the same health impact. Given the multiplicity of other factors that influence outcomes, the goal of the analysis will be to assess PEPFAR's *contribution* to changes in health impact, as direct *attribution* will not be possible.

- The evaluation will use a mixed methods approach to answer evaluation questions derived from the study charge and the guiding framework of the program impact pathway. By drawing on a combination of analytical techniques and on a range of both quantitative and qualitative data sources, the convergence among different findings will be assessed to support plausible conclusions about the effects or contributions of PEPFAR programs.

- The extent to which the evaluation goals can be met will depend on the timely availability of relevant data of sufficient quality. Many evaluation questions will require data that go beyond the indicators that are reported centrally to the Office of the U.S. Global AIDS Coordinator (OGAC). Data will have to be gathered from multiple sources, contingent upon the availability and feasibility of access within the timeframe of the evaluation.
    - The evaluation will draw on existing data and analyses as well as new data collection and new secondary analyses of existing data.
    - Data will be sought from OGAC and other U.S. government agencies; PEPFAR implementing partners; other bilateral and multilateral agencies and donors; country-level data from national governments, implementers, and the research community; the scientific health and development literature; and country studies, including document review and qualitative data collected from a select cross-section of PEPFAR countries during country visits conducted as part of the evaluation.

- The evaluation plan is designed with sufficient flexibility to adapt, to the extent possible, to the ongoing evolution of the PEPFAR program as well as to new policy issues, new information, and new sources of data that emerge as the evaluation itself proceeds.

- There will be limitations to the assessment due to the nature of the available data, the timing of the evaluation, and the distinct characteristics and complexities of each country in which the program operates.
    - Much of the data is not collected and/or reported systematically across PEPFAR. In most cases, the available data will be country-specific, implementing-partner-specific, or program component-specific. This will limit the ability to generalize or aggregate findings to the whole of the program, especially given the considerable heterogeneity in the implementation of PEPFAR across different countries and programs. However, with careful interpretation, the available data can inform conclusions that contribute to an understanding of the performance and impact of PEPFAR as a whole.
    - Some effects described in the statement of task, such as the impact on child mortality and on 5-year survival rates, will be particularly difficult to evaluate due to the limited available data that directly measure the desired outcome or impact. Instead, other measures and methods will be used to assess program effects on, for example, HIV incidence, outcomes for people living with HIV/AIDS, and child health.
    - It will be difficult to evaluate the impact of recent and imminent programmatic changes in response to the goals for shifting to a sustainable response because there will be insufficient time for these changes to be translated from implementation into measurable effects. However, the evaluation will assess efforts and process in these areas to provide insight into whether PEPFAR is making reasonable progress toward these new goals.

- Within the parameters of the evaluation design, the conclusions in the final report will focus on assessing the implementation and effects of program components and on providing guidance that aims to maximize the potential for programs to have a future positive health impact. Based on the conclusions of the evaluation, the IOM will make recommendations that focus on improving the U.S. government response to global HIV/AIDS, including support for and alignment with global and local responses at the country level. The recommendations will be intended to inform decisions about how to identify, disseminate, and scale up the most effective and efficient strategies in order to make the best use of limited resources to accomplish PEPFAR's evolving goals for a transition to a sustainable, country-owned response to the pandemic.

The evaluation described in this plan can be expected to contribute to the understanding of large-scale programmatic strategies to meet the needs of those living with HIV and AIDS and to prevent new HIV infections. The study will provide a rigorous, non-partisan, multidisciplinary, and independent evaluation of the PEPFAR program that will inform Congress and the Department of State, as well as the scientific community, program implementers, policy makers, civil society, people affected by HIV/AIDS, and international stakeholders in global public health.

# PART I

# Introduction and Background

# INTRODUCTION

## Epidemiology of the Pandemic

Since the first case was recognized in the early 1980's, the spread of the human immunodeficiency virus (HIV), which causes acquired immune deficiency syndrome (AIDS), has achieved pandemic proportions (CDC, 1981; UNAIDS, 2006). According to the latest report from the Joint United Nations Programme on HIV/AIDS (UNAIDS) and the World Health Organization (WHO) (2009), HIV/AIDS continues to be a major global health priority. In 2008, the number of people living with HIV worldwide reached an estimated 33 million, an increase of more than 20 percent since 2000 (UNAIDS and WHO, 2009). The number of new HIV infections in 2008 was estimated to be nearly 3 million, which is approximately 30 percent lower than at the pandemic's peak in 1996—with 84 percent of the new HIV infections occurring among people aged 15–49 years old (UNAIDS and WHO, 2009).

Sub-Saharan Africa accounts for 67 percent of people (approximately 22 million) living globally with HIV and continues to experience the greatest burden of the disease, including the largest proportion of new HIV infections in 2008. Asia follows with nearly 15 percent (approximately 5 million people) of adults and children living with HIV (UNAIDS and WHO, 2009). The Caribbean has the second highest adult HIV prevalence of 1 percent (UNAIDS and WHO, 2009). Worldwide, the prevalence of HIV reached peaks in the 1990s and early 2000s. The timing of peaks in incidence varied considerably, from the early 1980s to the mid 1990s, indicating that the peaks in incidence preceded those in prevalence by nearly a decade. This implies that prevalence continued to rise for a number of years after the incidence rate had begun to decline (UNAIDS and WHO, 2009).

The HIV pandemic is having an impact in every region of the world; some populations, however, demonstrate greater vulnerability to HIV infection. Several factors associated with this phenomenon are the major risks of drug use and sexual risk-taking behavior. These are also associated with poverty (or wealth in some countries), gender-based violence, access to health and education, culture and awareness about HIV, and stigma and discrimination. Discrimination and criminalization of behavior, for instance, may prevent groups such as men who have sex with men (MSM), injection drug users (IDU), and commercial sex workers (CSW) from accessing health care and other services in certain countries. Additional vulnerable sub-populations are women and girls, young people and children, out-of-school youth, and people affected or displaced by humanitarian crises (UNAIDS, 2010b). In sub-Saharan Africa, women and children are among the most vulnerable groups of the epidemic (WHO et al., 2009). Women account for nearly 60 percent of the estimated HIV infections in the region (UNAIDS, 2008), while young women aged 15–24 years old show on average three times the prevalence of their male counterparts in countries most affected by HIV/AIDS in southern Africa (Gouws et al., 2008). Despite the recent increase of antiretroviral therapy (ART) availability and coverage, HIV/AIDS remains a major cause of death worldwide—an estimated 2 million people died from AIDS in 2008—and AIDS remains a leading cause of death for people aged 15–49 years old in sub-Saharan Africa (UNAIDS and WHO, 2009). Furthermore, HIV/AIDS is the leading cause of death worldwide among women of reproductive age (WHO, 2009d)—globally there were approximately 16 million women living with HIV at the end of 2008 (UNAIDS and WHO, 2009).

To some extent, successful scale-up of ART has prolonged survival and resulted in growing numbers of people living with HIV infection (WHO et al., 2009). However, for every person placed on ART, even more people are becoming newly infected who need care and who may be potentially spreading infection. This leads to the concurrence that incident infections are outpacing the number of people placed on ART (Zachariah et al., 2010) and that implementation of effective prevention lags considerably.

Behind these numbers lies the broader impact of AIDS and associated diseases on populations and societies: plummeting life expectancy, changing population demographics (including a large impact in the working-age population group), and overloaded health systems. For instance, Swaziland experienced a dramatic reduction by half in average life expectancy between 1990 and 2007 (UNAIDS and WHO, 2009). Despite the expanded availability of HIV/AIDS services, the pandemic continues to affect the socioeconomic conditions of many of the least developed countries and requires continued commitment and support from not only the international community, but also the national governments of the affected countries (OGAC, 2009g). The primary challenges—and opportunities—facing the U.S. President's Emergency Plan for AIDS Relief (PEPFAR) in its current and future phases of operation are to facilitate sustainable country-driven responses to the pandemic that reduce HIV incidence, are commensurate with the needs of people living with HIV, and strengthen health systems to better address HIV-related health needs.

## Organization of the Report

This report is organized into three principal parts. Part I describes the epidemiology of the HIV/AIDS pandemic, key information from the original and reauthorizing legislation for the U.S. global HIV/AIDS initiative, the strategies for program implementation under this U.S. initiative, and some organizational information for the office that administers these HIV/AIDS programs. It also describes the first congressionally mandated study for the U.S. Institute of Medicine (IOM) to evaluate the implementation of the HIV/AIDS programs under the initiative. Following the introduction and background, Part II describes the proposed evaluation approach, including methodologies and data sources, for the new congressionally mandated IOM evaluation of the same programs from 2004–2011. In particular, the evaluation approach is organized around a program impact pathway based on a theory of change model that identifies the intermediate steps between the inputs invested in the program and the ultimate impact on health. Part III applies this model of change to specific parts of PEPFAR in response to the legislative directive for the evaluation. It provides descriptions and presents illustrative evaluation questions that will be used to guide the evaluation of the performance and impact of specific programmatic areas as well as other key systems level goals such as health systems strengthening and transitioning to sustainability

## BACKGROUND

### The U.S. Leadership Against HIV/AIDS, Tuberculosis, and Malaria Act

In his 2003 State of the Union address, President Bush proposed that the U.S. Congress authorize $15 billion, over 5 years, to globally address HIV/AIDS—making the proposed health initiative the largest single donor investment for a single disease in U.S. history (Bush, 2003).

The U.S. Congress' authorization of the U.S. Leadership Against HIV/AIDS, Tuberculosis, and Malaria Act of 2003 (the Leadership Act)[1] marked an important contribution to the global response to HIV/AIDS, including the commitment of significant new funding and attention. Before the establishment of the PEPFAR program, however, the U.S. Government (USG) was already making significant investments to combat HIV and AIDS in developing countries. The United States Agency for International Development's (USAID) HIV/AIDS funding grew from $1.1 million in fiscal year (FY) 1986 to $433 million in FY2001 (USAID, 2009b). On July 19, 1999, the Clinton Administration launched a $100 million initiative called Leadership and Investment in Fighting an Epidemic. This initiative supported the increase of funding to address the global AIDS pandemic by focusing on primary prevention, care and treatment, as well as capacity and infrastructure development (USAID, 2000). A Kaiser Family Foundation report on bilateral donations from 15 donor countries in 1996 and 1997 placed the United States as the largest donor of HIV/AIDS official donor assistance, contributing 49 percent of the total amount (Alagiri et al., 2001). In 2002, President Bush launched the $500 million International Mother and Child HIV Prevention Initiative with a goal of preventing mother-to-child transmission by up to 40 percent. Activities were directed to support expansion of national prevention of mother-to-child transmission (PMTCT) programs and linkage of PMTCT services with ART and care for mothers, infants, and family members, with a target of reaching up to 1 million women annually in 12 African and 2 Caribbean countries with high rates of HIV/AIDS. These activities and countries, which were to become the "focus countries" (Vietnam was later added), were subsumed as a major activity under PEPFAR and were coordinated across several USG agencies including the Centers for Disease Control and Prevention (CDC) and USAID (CRS, 2003; KFF, 2009; Shaffer et al., 2004).

The Leadership Act required (1) the President to establish a comprehensive, integrated Five-Year Strategy to combat global HIV/AIDS focusing on prevention, treatment and care strategies; (2) the assignment of priorities for pertinent executive branches; (3) better coordination mechanisms among such agencies; (4) the provision of the resources needed to achieve the projected goals; and (5) the coordination of provided resources with related assistance from multilateral organizations, other international organizations, governments of foreign countries, and appropriate governmental and non-governmental organizations (NGO). A specific emphasis was given to programs based on women and children's vulnerabilities, to support the development of countries' health care infrastructure and human resources, and to periodic monitoring and evaluation (M&E).

In addition, the legislation created the position of the U.S. Global AIDS Coordinator (the Coordinator) within the U.S. Department of State (DoS) with the rank of ambassador. The Coordinator would be appointed by the President, with advice and consent of the Senate, and would be accountable for the oversight and coordination of all U.S. international resources and efforts to fight the HIV/AIDS pandemic. Ambassador Randall Tobias was sworn in as the first Coordinator (2003–2006) and presented the first required Five-Year Global HIV/AIDS Strategy to Congress on February 2004. Ambassador Mark R. Dybul succeeded Tobias (2006–2009), and currently Ambassador Eric Goosby serves as the Coordinator.

---

[1] United States Leadership against HIV/AIDS, Tuberculosis, and Malaria Act of 2003, P.L.108-25, 108th Cong.,1st Sess. (May 27, 2003).

## The President's Emergency Plan for AIDS Relief

The title given to the U.S. Five-Year Global HIV/AIDS Strategy, "The U.S. President's Emergency Plan for AIDS Relief," or PEPFAR, became the common name for the program (hereinafter referred to as PEPFAR I). PEPFAR I's strategy established three overarching goals to guide the development of the initiative: (1) to encourage bold leadership at every level to fight HIV/AIDS; (2) to apply best practices within bilateral HIV/AIDS prevention, treatment, and care programs, in concert with the objectives and policies of partner governments' national HIV/AIDS strategies; and (3) to encourage partners, including multilateral organizations and other partner governments, to coordinate at all levels to strengthen response efforts, to embrace best practices, to adhere to principles of sound management, and to harmonize monitoring M&E efforts to ensure the most effective and efficient use of resources (IOM, 2007). The principles for achieving the stated goals were emphasized in the initial strategy as well, including responding with urgency to the crisis; seeking new approaches; establishing and ensuring accountability for measurable goals; harmonizing program development and implementation with the partner countries; integrating prevention, treatment, and care programs; and building national capacity (OGAC, 2004).

PEPFAR I's funding (from 2004 to 2008) was focused on establishing and scaling up prevention, care, and treatment programs, and reaching specific performance targets of preventing 7 million new HIV infections by 2010, treating 2 million HIV-infected people with antiretroviral (ARV) drugs by 2008, and providing care for 10 million people infected with and affected by HIV/AIDS (including orphans and vulnerable children) by 2008. Two-thirds of the originally funded $15 billion was directed to be appropriated to 15 "focus" countries,[2] selected because their HIV/AIDS burden represented, at the time, at least 50 percent of global HIV prevalence. Budgetary targets for the program included 55 percent to be spent on treatment for individuals with HIV/AIDS, 20 percent for the prevention of HIV/AIDS (with at least a third of that money going to programs that promoted only abstinence and being faithful), 15 percent for palliative care of infected individuals, and 10 percent for orphans and vulnerable children (IOM, 2007). Less intense activities were also performed in more than 120 countries with the remainder of the funding (IOM, 2007).

## The Office of the U.S. Global AIDS Coordinator

*Headquarters Level*

The administrative office and formal organizational unit for PEPFAR is the Office of the Global AIDS Coordinator (OGAC) at the DoS. Overseen by the Coordinator, it directs activities at both the headquarters level in Washington, DC, and at the country level in the designated PEPFAR countries[3] under the additional oversight of the U.S. Ambassador of the country.

---

[2] The 15 focus countries included Botswana, Republic of Côte d'Ivoire, Federal Democratic Republic of Ethiopia, Cooperative Republic of Guyana, Republic of Haiti, Republic of Kenya, Republic of Mozambique, Republic of Namibia, Federal Republic of Nigeria, Republic of Rwanda, Republic of South Africa, United Republic of Tanzania, Republic of Uganda, Socialist Republic of Vietnam, and Republic of Zambia.

[3] The current PEPFAR countries include the following additions to the original 15 focus countries: Republic of Angola, Kingdom of Cambodia, People's Republic of China, Democratic Republic of the Congo, Dominican Republic, Republic of Ghana, Republic of India, Republic of Indonesia, Kingdom of Lesotho, Republic of Malawi,

OGAC staff, including detailees of other USG agencies, are organized into numerous divisions including Executive Director, Management and Budget, New Partner Outreach, Public-Private Partnerships, Strategic Information, Multilateral Diplomacy, and Program Services. OGAC also has a Chief of Staff and Legal Advisor, as well as liaisons for Congressional Relations, and Public Affairs and Public Diplomacy (see Figure 1).

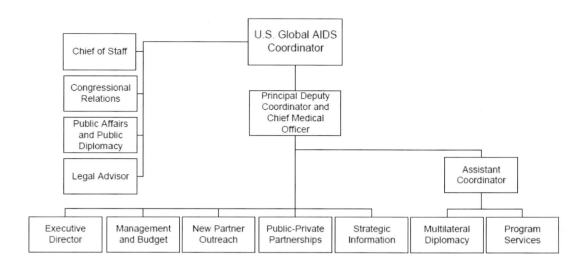

**Office of the U.S. Global AIDS Coordinator**
President's Emergency Plan for AIDS Relief

**FIGURE 1** Organizational structure of OGAC (last updated October 16, 2007).
SOURCE: PEPFAR (2007).

Guidance also is provided by the Agency Principals and the administrative heads of the agencies involved in implementing PEPFAR programs.[4] Additional advisory bodies and processes provide assistance to OGAC for information sharing and decision making for programmatic activities. For example, USG agency program directors form the Deputy Principals, who advise political appointees in the Principals group and the AIDS Coordinator on programmatic and policy guidance. There are Country and Regional Support Teams. Other technical advisory bodies for headquarters include the Technical Working Groups (TWGs)[5] that

---

Russian Federation, Republic of the Sudan, Kingdom of Swaziland, Kingdom of Thailand, and the Ukraine (personal communication from OGAC, June 16, 2009).
[4] The Department of Defense; Department of Health and Human Services including CDC, Health Resources and Services Administration, Food and Drug Administration, National Institutes of Health, Substance Abuse and Mental Health Services Administration; Department of Labor; Department of Commerce; DoS; the Peace Corps; and USAID (IOM, 2007).
[5] OGAC operates the following TWGs (by program area): General population sexual prevention, Most-At-Risk Persons, Medical Transmission, Counseling and Testing, Prevention with Positives, Male Circumcision Taskforce, Human Resources for Health, Adult Treatment, PMTCT/Pediatric AIDS, Community/Faith Based Organizations, Tuberculosis (TB) and HIV/AIDS, Orphans and Vulnerable Children, Care and Support, Food and Nutrition, Public-Private Partnerships, Strategic Information, Gender, Laboratory. Staff from USG agencies, USG-funded partners, and non-USG-funded partners may participate in each TWG (Personal communication from OGAC, June 16, 2009).

provide programmatic guidance by service area and topic, the USG Global Fund Technical Support Advisory Panel, and the Technical Advisory Board (TAB). The TAB was instituted by the Deputy Principals to support their work with the TWGs, provide technical assistance and policy recommendations to the Deputy Principals, and provide overarching coordination and function of the TWGs. In 2009, the TAB presented its analysis of the work of the TWGs called the State of the Program Areas, in which it identified promising practices, gaps in programming, and accomplishments of the TWGs (Stanton, 2009). The primary function of the TAB is to inform the Deputy Principals of policy considerations for upcoming program planning.

*Country Level*

At the country level, each country that was formerly a focus country has a U.S. Country Team, which coordinates all the program activities. By 2009, the 16 additional countries and regions were also building interagency HIV/AIDS teams and submitting a country operational plan (COP) to OGAC. Although implementation may vary depending on the needs and capacity of the country, the general structure of the program is intended to be similar across countries. The U.S. Ambassador ensures policy and program coordination at the highest levels and assures accountability for all reports and plans submitted to OGAC. The staff of the Country Teams include representatives from all the implementing departments and agencies. Each Team is anchored by a Country Coordinator located within the U.S. embassy (see Figure 2). Chiefs of Mission provide essential leadership to interagency HIV/AIDS teams and, along with other U.S. officials, engage in policy discussions with partner-country leaders to generate additional attention and resources for the pandemic and ensure strong partner coordination. The activities support the performance targets in prevention, treatment, and care, as well as other areas, such as M&E, capacity building, developing partnership frameworks, and health systems strengthening.

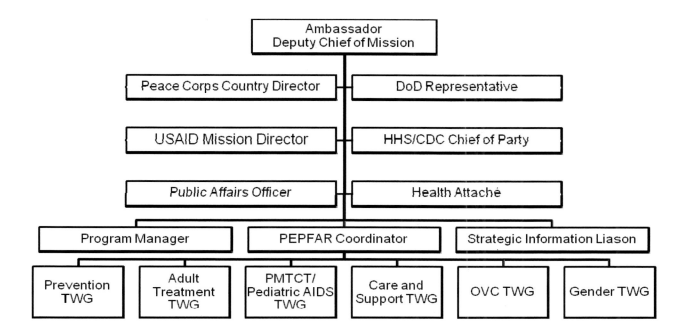

**FIGURE 2** Model structure of PEPFAR Country Teams.
NOTE: The structure of each team will vary by country. Different TWGs are present in different countries, and this figure includes an illustrative example. CDC = U.S. Centers for Disease Control and Prevention, DoD = U.S. Department of Defense, HHS = U.S. Department of Health and Human Services, OVC = orphans and vulnerable children, PMTCT = prevention of mother-to-child transmission, TWG = technical working groups, USAID = United States Agency for International Development.
SOURCE: Adapted from personal communications from OGAC (June 16, 2009).

## IOM's First Evaluation of PEPFAR: "PEPFAR Implementation: Progress and Promise"

In accordance with the Leadership Act mandate, the IOM evaluated the implementation of PEPFAR three years after the program's authorization to provide a final report in 2007 as guidance for Congress for its consideration of reauthorization of the program. The IOM focused this evaluation on the initial implementation of PEPFAR in the 15 focus countries. The evaluation, due to logistical constraints, was not an impact assessment and did not include the U.S. contribution to the Global Fund to Fight AIDS, Tuberculosis, and Malaria (Global Fund) (IOM, 2005). The study was planned, designed, and conducted by an independent expert committee with three subcommittees convened by the IOM and several consultants (IOM, 2007).

The framework developed for the first evaluation set the concept of "harmonization" at the center of the plan, focusing the evaluation on the contribution of PEPFAR I to the development of countries' capacity to address their HIV/AIDS epidemics. This was based on the "Three Ones," principles endorsed by many international donors and United Nations agencies. These guiding principles of harmonization—one agreed HIV/AIDS Action Framework, one National HIV/AIDS Coordinating Authority, and one agreed HIV/AIDS country-level M&E system—were intended to improve the country-level HIV/AIDS response, and reduce the transactional costs of business between countries and multiple donors (UNAIDS, 2004).

A wide range of methods was used, including six information-gathering and deliberative meetings; review of the scientific and other literature; review of PEPFAR and other documentation; and discussions with PEPFAR staff, in-country implementation partners, and other donors and stakeholders. The committee also analyzed PEPFAR I's budget and program performance data. Although it did not independently audit or verify these data, it did some checks for internal consistency as well as congruence with external sources (IOM, 2007).

The committee visited 13 of the 15 focus countries in small delegations between late October of 2005 and late February of 2006. Due to security concerns, the committee was unable to visit Côte d'Ivoire and Haiti, but conducted several conference calls with the Country Teams and implementing partners (IOM, 2007). The country visits were used to directly observe implementation activities, but did not review the details of all the programs funded by PEPFAR I. Each IOM country team rendered a report with the summary of the consensus on the key observations, findings, and conclusions about PEPFAR I activities in that particular country. This information was also used to reach conclusions across the focus countries using several types of analyses. The committee "triangulated" these syntheses of information from the focus countries with other sources of information—including documentation and other interviews—to reach conclusions about key aspects of PEPFAR I implementation, such as harmonization (IOM, 2007).

According to the first IOM evaluation, PEPFAR made progress toward meeting the performance targets of PEPFAR I in the first 2 years and established a foundation for achieving the broader, longer-term goals of the Leadership Act. The committee placed emphasis on the need to transition from an emergency response to one of sustainability to achieve these longer-term goals. PEPFAR was also identified as a functioning learning organization in many areas, including research efforts, communications, knowledge dissemination and contributions to the global evidence base to address HIV/AIDS, and quality improvement to facilitate building capacity to support the transition. The committee stated that PEPFAR would benefit from developing a detailed strategy to institutionalize the concept of being a learning organization that would also enable tracking and reporting of progress toward goals of the strategy (IOM, 2007). However, that report also identified the continuing challenge of supporting a substantial expansion of HIV/AIDS services, while placing greater efforts on long-term strategic planning and the development of countries' capacity building for sustainability (IOM, 2007).

The main recommendations from the first IOM evaluation were categorized in three groups: (1) the need to address long-term factors, such as expanding prevention strategies, improving the status of vulnerable groups such as women and girls, building workforce capacity, and increasing the knowledge base by means of publishing research conducted; (2) the need to improve harmonization with international and national stakeholders, providing support to the WHO on their drug prequalification process, and removing budget allocations or "earmarks" associated with performance targets; and (3) the need to expand, improve, and integrate services based on evidence-based strategies and exhausting the existing local capacity, providing adequate medications for treatment, using community-based care, establishing performance targets for orphans and vulnerable children and addressing the needs of marginalized populations.

### Tom Lantos and Henry J. Hyde United States Global Leadership Against HIV/AIDS, Tuberculosis, and Malaria Reauthorization Act of 2008

On July 30, 2008, the U.S. Congress passed the Tom Lantos and Henry J. Hyde United States Global Leadership Against HIV/AIDS, Tuberculosis, and Malaria Reauthorization Act of 2008 (hereinafter, the Lantos–Hyde Act of 2008).[6] The primary goal of this reauthorization legislation was to continue the USG commitment to the program for 5 additional years, from 2009 through 2013 (hereinafter referred to as PEPFAR II), authorizing up to $39 billion exclusively for PEPFAR bilateral HIV/AIDS programs and U.S. contributions to the Global Fund. New cumulative performance targets for 2013 under the Lantos–Hyde Act of 2008 include preventing 12 million new infections worldwide (without a proportional goal stated for women or children), providing care for 12 million people living with or affected by HIV/AIDS including 5 million orphans and other children made vulnerable due to HIV/AIDS, and training and retaining at least 140,000 new health care workers.[7] In addition, the reauthorization legislation supports the increase in the number of individuals with HIV/AIDS receiving ART above two million people, which was the initial goal under the Leadership Act of 2003. The Lantos–Hyde Act of 2008 also eliminated nearly all of the fiscal benchmarks established in the original legislation, with the exception of the 10 percent target for orphans and vulnerable children and the treatment earmark directing that at least half of funds must be spent on ART and other treatment services. Additionally, there are new programmatic requirements, many related to prevention activities, which are discussed in the section on prevention in Part III of this report.

In December 2009, Ambassador Goosby issued a new PEPFAR Five-Year Strategy, which includes the targets in the reauthorization legislation, but specified the treatment target of providing direct support for more than 4 million people (OGAC, 2009g). However, different from the legislation, the strategic plan extends the time frame of these cumulative performance targets through FY2014 (OGAC, 2009g). Furthermore, the new PEPFAR Five-Year Strategy defined the future direction of PEPFAR II and clearly established the need to (1) transition from an emergency response to promoting sustainable country programs; (2) strengthen partner government capacity to lead the response to this epidemic and other health demands; (3) expand prevention, care, and treatment in both concentrated and generalized epidemics; (4) integrate and coordinate HIV/AIDS programs with broader global health and development programs to maximize impact on health systems; and (5) invest in innovation and operations research to evaluate impact, improve service delivery, and maximize outcomes (OGAC, 2009g).

This strategy also describes how PEPFAR can help leverage additional investments in global health as a part of the Obama Administration's new $63 billion,[8] 6-year Global Health Initiative (GHI) (OGAC, 2009h). The Initiative's consultation document indicates how it will incorporate PEPFAR's strategic cumulative goals within a comprehensive U.S. global health policy approach that will focus attention on broader global health challenges (DoS, 2010b). Although this evaluation will not focus on the targets or activities for the GHI beyond PEPFAR, summary information on the initiative is in Box 1.

---

[6] Tom Lantos and Henry J. Hyde United States Global Leadership Against HIV/AIDS, Tuberculosis, and Malaria Reauthorization Act of 2008, Public Law 110-293, 110th Cong., 2nd sess. (July 30, 2008).

[7] *Ibid.*, §301(a)(2), 22 U.S.C. §2151b-2(b)(1)(A).

[8] This amount includes the funds for the second operational phase of PEPFAR (2009–2013) and other international health programs.

---

**BOX 1**
**PEPFAR and the U.S. Global Health Initiative**

In May 2009, President Barack Obama announced a new U.S. government (USG) Global Health Initiative (GHI). In February 2010, an implementation plan was published as a consultation document to outline a core focus to improve health outcomes in low-income countries through strengthened platforms and systems and utilization of a new business model for USG global health assistance. The GHI expands beyond HIV/AIDS to enhance the focus on other areas, particularly maternal and child health, family planning and reproductive health, and neglected tropical diseases. As the largest bilateral health assistance program of the USG, PEPFAR is expected to be an integral foundation for the GHI. As with PEPFAR, the transition to strengthened, integrated, and sustained health systems owned and driven by country priorities is considered a centerpiece. This will necessitate a re-orientation "away from parallel systems to more concerted support for national health systems" (OGAC, 2009h, p. 27). Commitment is also signalled for short- and long-term measurement of quality, outcomes, cost-effectiveness, innovation, and impact. The need to improve government accountability and to provide financial and program management technical assistance to support these activities is acknowledged. Human resource planning and health professional pre-service education, task-shifting, retention, and re-employment models also are essential components of the GHI.

In its most recent budget request for fiscal year (FY) 2011, the Administration proposed to designate $200 million in funding for up to 20 "GHI Plus" country partners (10 in FY2011–2012 and 10 in FY2013) of which $100 million is slated to come from Department of State funding (the other $100 million will come from other United States Agency for International Development (USAID) global health programs). The GHI will encourage operational research, considering evaluation, program learning, innovation, and dissemination as key to the Initiative's success.

SOURCES: DoS (2010a, 2010b); OGAC (2009h).

# PART II

# Proposed Evaluation Approach

# CONGRESSIONAL CHARGE AND PLANNING PHASE APPROACH

Under the Lantos–Hyde Act of 2008,[9] Congress mandated that the IOM conduct a study that includes an assessment of the performance of U.S.-assisted global HIV/AIDS programs and an evaluation of the impact on health of prevention, treatment, and care efforts that are supported by U.S. funding, including multilateral and bilateral programs involving joint operations (see Appendix A). Based on clarifications with congressional staff and OGAC,[10] the charge is intended to focus on the performance and impact of bilaterally funded PEPFAR programs in the current partner countries (see Table 1 in Part III, Section 2 for a list of countries). This will include programs and activities that are operated jointly with both bilateral funding through PEPFAR and funding through the Global Fund. Consistent with the clarified congressional intent, U.S. contributions to the Global Fund that are not a part of activities *jointly* funded or implemented by PEPFAR will not be the focus of the evaluation, and the evaluation will not compare the performance of bilateral PEPFAR programs to that of Global Fund programs (Bressler, 2009; Marsh, 2009). The study will consider PEPFAR's performance and impact since funding first became available in 2004. The timing of the study, with a final report to be delivered in 2012, dictates that the evaluation will consider data that are now, or will become, available through 2011.

As the first phase of this study, the IOM was charged to form an ad hoc committee to develop a strategic plan for the assessment and evaluation of HIV/AIDS programs implemented under the Lantos–Hyde Act of 2008 and to issue a short report to the U.S. Congress describing the plan's proposed design, taking into consideration the requirements for the congressionally mandated study. These requirements and the charge for developing the evaluation plan can be found in full in the Statement of Task in Appendix A. More information about the members of the planning committee can be found in Appendix B. This report documenting the proposed evaluation approach is the product for the first phase of the study.

To produce this report, the planning committee met three times to deliberate in person, conducted two teleconferences, and engaged in additional deliberations in smaller working groups by telephonic and electronic communications as needed. In the development of its plan, the committee consulted widely, and remains open to receiving input from, the broad range of parties interested in and affected by PEPFAR. To solicit input and gather information from a wide range of stakeholders, public sessions were held in conjunction with the first and second committee meetings, and delegations from the committee and IOM project staff also held information-gathering meetings with a range of global stakeholders, including UNAIDS, WHO, the United Nations Children's Fund (UNICEF), and the Global Fund. The primary purpose of these meetings was to establish working relationships with these stakeholders and to discuss potential data sources and methodologies, as well as strategies and lessons learned from large-scale programmatic or organizational evaluations. The agendas for these activities can be found in Appendix C. In addition, one staff member attended the PEPFAR Annual Implementers' Meeting in 2009. The committee also consulted the available literature on PEPFAR, global HIV/AIDS, and the state of the art in large-scale program evaluation, including the summary of a

---

[9] *Supra.*, note 6 at §101(c), 22 U.S.C. 7611(c).
[10] Personal communications from Congressional Staff at the U.S. House Committee on Foreign Affairs and U.S. Senate Committee on Foreign Relations and OGAC, 2009.

workshop convened by the IOM, "Design Considerations for Evaluating the Impact of PEPFAR," which focused on methodological, policy, and practical considerations (IOM, 2008).

The committee and staff also conducted an initial scan of potential data sources for the forthcoming evaluation using a range of sources, including a preliminary review of documents from OGAC and other bilateral and multilateral agencies and of relevant published literature, as well as communications with a wide range of staff from OGAC, implementing partners, and multilateral stakeholders. The committee used this information to assess the methods that could be employed to answer evaluation questions based on the charge in the statement of task, focusing on data and methodology that will be robust, available, feasible, and appropriate to the questions. Through this information gathering and deliberation, the planning committee developed a conceptual framework for the evaluation that is based on both the committee's expertise and current standards in evaluation methodologies for large-scale programs.

This report is intended to provide Congress and OGAC with an overview of the strategic plan for the forthcoming evaluation. As agreed upon contractually with the study sponsor, the planning process for the evaluation will culminate with a transitional period for operational planning that will take place between the delivery of this report and the implementation of the evaluation itself in the fall of 2010. During this operational planning phase, IOM staff, planning committee members, and consultants will carry out activities to further develop and refine the plan described here. These activities, which will inform the implementation of the evaluation, are described as part of the work plan later in this section. This structure for the study, with a report describing strategic elements of the plan delivered to Congress before detailed operational planning is complete, was intentionally designed to allow uninterrupted progress in preparation for the evaluation during the time necessary for review of the report and budget planning by the sponsor and for subsequent preparation of the contract for the evaluation.

After congressional review of the plan's proposed design and budget, the final phase of the project will be to carry out the assessment/evaluation of the program. The IOM will convene a new ad-hoc committee to conduct the evaluation as a consensus study. The intent is for the evaluation committee and staff to have considerable overlap from the planning committee. Standard IOM procedures will be followed to ensure that the evaluation committee and project staff have the appropriate expertise to conduct the evaluation activities described in this report.

## EVALUATION GOALS AND CONCEPTUAL FRAMEWORK FOR EVALUATION DESIGN

The legislative mandate to evaluate PEPFAR is a complex challenge. As described above, PEPFAR is a large, multifaceted program with many activities carried out by many different partners in a diverse group of countries. In addition, PEPFAR activities are being implemented in the context of programs supported by other funders that have the same ultimate aim. PEPFAR is also by necessity a dynamic program; the ability to change the program over time can be beneficial, but makes evaluation difficult as it presents a "moving target." Therefore, this report not only outlines an approach for evaluating the performance of PEPFAR, but also delineates the challenges in evaluating the impact of such a complex, large-scale foreign assistance program and provides information about reasonable and appropriate expectations for an evaluation of this kind. The committee has endeavored to present a plan that is thorough and well-defined in its approach yet maintains ample flexibility. This will allow the evaluation to be adapted in response both to the evolving goals of the program and to the additional information the evaluation committee will gather during operational planning and as the evaluation itself proceeds.

The proposed conceptual framework for the evaluation and its limitations will be described briefly here, followed by a more thorough discussion of the methods and data sources that will be used. The subsequent sections in Part III of this report address specific components of the evaluation in greater detail.

## Evaluation Goals and Assumptions

The planning committee understood the mandate from Congress as a charge to develop a plan to assess the program with two primary goals. The first of these is an assessment of the success of the program in meeting the performance goals and targets laid out in two sources: the reauthorization legislation and the new PEPFAR Five-Year Strategy. Although the statement of task was written before the new strategic plan was available, the committee interpreted the charge to take this document into account because it articulates the current guiding principles and the future direction for the program. Therefore, the evaluation will include a careful review and comparison of these guiding documents in order to more clearly define the targets and goals of the program. The second goal of the committee's charge is to evaluate the health impact of PEPFAR, including impact of treatment, care, and prevention programs; effects on health systems; efforts to address gender-specific aspects of HIV/AIDS; impact of programs on child mortality; and impact of interventions on behalf of orphans and vulnerable children. The findings and conclusions of the evaluation of PEPFAR's progress toward its stated goals and the impact of the program will then be used to make recommendations for improving the USG response to global HIV/AIDS, in particular through PEPFAR programs.

It is important to note that the IOM is being charged to conduct an evaluation early in the implementation of changes to the program in response to the reauthorization legislation and the new PEPFAR Five-Year Strategy. These changes reflect a progressive transition to a new era of challenges and goals for the program, which include efforts to improve sustainability of the response over time, to enhance coordination with partner governments and other global funding partners, and to support accountable ownership of HIV program delivery by countries themselves. They also reflect efforts to give greater consideration to the relationship of PEPFAR to broader health and development needs in partner countries. The timing of this evaluation, with data collection extending through 2011 for a final report due in 2012, will make it difficult to evaluate the outcomes or impact of these most recent changes so soon after implementation. For example, it could take several years or even decades for a full effect to be realized from some efforts to strengthen health systems, such as the training and retention of new health care workers or the strengthening of health information systems to support M&E efforts. However, the evaluation will assess efforts, process, and initial results in these areas to provide insight into whether PEPFAR is making reasonable progress toward these new goals and to lead to recommendations for how the program can be improved to ensure that these evolving goals for the program can be met. As part of this, the evaluation will assess whether there is sufficient M&E capacity in place to eventually evaluate whether the program has met these goals as well as the resulting outcomes and impact.

The legislative mandate calls for the assessment of PEPFAR to be delivered in 2012; this would coincide with reauthorization discussions for the program, which the current legislation extends through 2013. It is of course not possible to predict the future needs and priorities of

Congress and OGAC with complete accuracy, but the planning committee's goal was to design an evaluation approach that, to the extent possible, looks ahead to anticipate the evolution of the program and therefore produce findings that address key issues under consideration at the time of the report release, including discussions about possible future legislative reauthorization.

### Conceptual Framework for Evaluation Design

The planning committee developed an overall conceptual framework for the evaluation, which calls for the use of a program impact pathway to guide an assessment of the contribution of PEPFAR to changes in health impact within the context of multiple international and national funding streams. This program impact pathway, described in more detail below, illustrates the committee's understanding of how PEPFAR programs are currently structured and intended to ultimately translate into health impacts, laying out a plausible pathway for causal effects. It represents the theory of change that underlies the program—in other words, the rationale for how the combination of activities supported by PEPFAR are logically expected to produce intermediate outcomes, which are then expected to collectively contribute, along with programs funded by other sources, to the desired population health impact. The use of a program impact pathway, which is also referred to as a logic model or results chain, has become well established as a method for evaluating complex, large-scale development assistance programs and is becoming widely accepted as a standard in the global HIV/AIDS community (Leeuw and Vaessen, 2009; UNAIDS MERG, 2010).[11]

Guided by the program impact pathway, the evaluation committee will use a mixed methods approach that will draw on a combination of analytical techniques and on a range of both quantitative and qualitative data sources. By assessing whether there is convergence and consistency among different data sources and methods, the evaluation committee will seek to triangulate findings that support reasonable, plausible linkages to outcomes and impact (Greene et al., 1989; Leeuw and Vaessen, 2009). The methods and data in the mix will complement each other, and will each have different strengths and limitations. This approach helps to account for the reality that, even given access to all potential data sources and extensive evaluation resources, there still would not be direct measures to answer many of the evaluation questions posed in the charge to the IOM. However, when taken together, the totality of evidence will allow the evaluation committee to draw conclusions and make recommendations for the program as a whole.

### *Program Impact Pathway*

Figure 3 shows the program impact pathway that the planning committee developed to represent a plausible causal chain of results for PEPFAR. The pathway begins with a series of investments or inputs to the program. For PEPFAR, these inputs include not only funding and other resources but also strategic planning, programmatic and policy guidance, technical assistance, and knowledge transfer and research that represent the evolving evidence base. These inputs support activities that provide services and support to children, adolescents, and adults in need. Although these services are described by PEPFAR in categories like prevention, treatment,

---

[11] Many of the terms used in the program impact pathway have different meanings in different fields of research. In this report, the terms correspond to definitions that reflect the current consensus in program evaluation. Definitions can be found in the glossary (Appendix D).

and care and support, the conceptual framework acknowledges that they are all part of an interrelated and overlapping approach, which also includes activities around gender issues and capacity building. These activities result in outputs that are measureable proximal effects. When the program is implemented well, these outputs are expected to produce outcomes as intermediate effects on the pathway to the ultimate goal of health impact. These intermediate outcomes include, for example, the delivery of high-quality, efficient services that are available and accessible to the targeted populations and that are achieving the intended and appropriate coverage. Other target outcomes include, for example, health systems strengthening; changes in individual risk behavior; and changes in knowledge, norms, and attitudes that affect sexual behavior, stigma, and gender issues. Ultimately, the program is intended to operate through this pathway to contribute to an impact on individual and population health and well-being, including HIV incidence, HIV prevalence, morbidity, and mortality.

Data will not be available to directly measure all of the outcomes and impacts illustrated in the impact pathway, and when available may need to come from sources other than PEPFAR. In some cases, such as assessing effects on incidence, proxy measures or modeling data will have to be used. A critical advantage of the program impact pathway approach is that it identifies the intermediate steps between the inputs invested in the program and the ultimate impact on health. This allows the evaluation to consider not just the beginning and endpoints, but also to assess whether the program is performing in the way it is intended along the full range of its implementation. Thus, even when it is not possible to assess impact directly, the evaluation committee will be able to state plausible findings about the effects of the program and draw conclusions that provide more refined and useful information about elements of the program that are functioning well or that could be improved in order to result in a greater impact on health.

For each of the programmatic areas that will be assessed in the evaluation, the committee will work from more specific program impact pathways. These are described in Part III of this report, along with illustrative evaluation questions based on the committee's interpretation of its charge to assess PEPFAR's performance and impact. All of the specific program impact pathways are oriented to describe outcomes that contribute to the HIV-related health impacts shown in Figure 3, which represent the stated overall goals of PEPFAR.

*24*

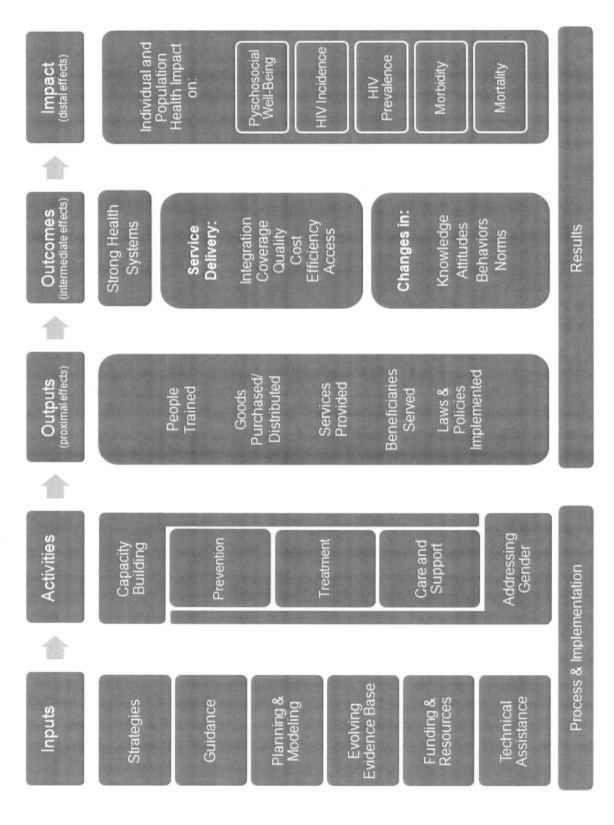

**FIGURE 3** Program impact pathway for evaluation of PEPFAR's effects on HIV-related health impact for children and adults. In the case of joint PEPFAR and Global Fund programs, some inputs may be provided by the Global Fund.

Although it provides a critical guide for developing evaluation questions, assessing data sources, and selecting methodologies, the program impact pathway is of course a simplified view of PEPFAR programs and their impact. Of particular importance for this evaluation's conceptual framework is the reality that in any country that receives PEPFAR support, the program operates within the context of a wide range of other factors that affect the implementation of the program as well as health outcomes (see Figure 4). Investments from a range of other sources support programs that are aimed at the same desired outcomes, and the proportion of total HIV/AIDS support that is provided by PEPFAR varies from country to country. In some cases, multiple funding sources may be co-mingled to support the same programs. Therefore, changes in population health that can be used to reflect program impact cannot be separated by specific programs or investments. Even individual measures can be difficult to attribute directly, as an individual or household may be receiving different services from different programs funded through different sources, all of which have an impact on the health outcomes of the beneficiary. Health outcomes are also influenced by a wide range of cultural, societal, geographical, and political factors and influences that the program cannot control. In addition, as PEPFAR programs increasingly operate with an emphasis on country ownership and harmonization with national plans, the extent to which central USG guidance and authority can influence all levels of priority-setting, decision making, and implementation can be quite limited. Finally, with a foreign assistance program that is implemented as broadly and on the scale of PEPFAR, there is rarely an appropriate comparison available in order to attribute outcomes to the program based on what would have happened in the absence of the investment.

Therefore, although the ideal goal in a program impact assessment may be to determine to what extent a desired outcome can be attributed directly to the program or policy investment, the realities of a large-scale program such as PEPFAR can make it difficult to determine the extent to which successes or failures in achieving the intended effect can be attributed directly to the program. Thus, the aim of this proposed evaluation approach is not to attempt to determine the direct attribution of PEPFAR funds to health outcomes. Rather, the aim is to assess the plausible contribution of PEPFAR to changes in health impact, both globally and by country, within the landscape of broader funding, programs, and other factors that influence health. This contribution analysis approach is consistent with the guidance given to the committee by congressional staff about expectations for the evaluation (Bressler, 2009; Marsh, 2009). It is also accepted as an appropriate standard for large-scale development assistance programs (Leeuw and Vaessen, 2009).

There may be some areas in which attribution can be more readily determined or approximated, as in the direct relationship at the first step of the impact pathway between inputs and the activities they support, or in the case of controlled experimental studies that assess the effects of intervention components that are distinct to PEPFAR, or in countries where PEPFAR is or has been the nearly exclusive funder of all national HIV/AIDS activities. If feasible, when these opportunities arise, the evaluation committee will consider whether a finding of attribution may be plausible.

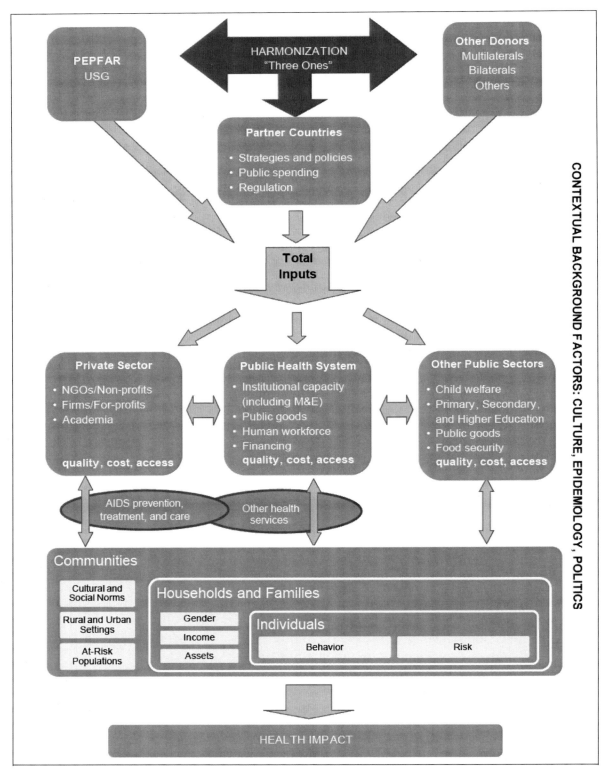

**FIGURE 4** Context for PEPFAR program implementation.
NOTES: M&E = monitoring and evaluation; USG = U.S. government; NGOs = non-governmental organizations.

## OVERARCHING EVALUATION CHALLENGES AND LIMITATIONS

There are a number of overarching challenges to carrying out this evaluation. These are described here, while more specific challenges and limitations are described in more detail in the following sections on evaluation methodologies and data sources as well as in the subsequent sections in Part III of this report that address specific components of the evaluation.

One of the primary challenges to the evaluation is that there are limited data to address health impact and other evaluation questions about the whole of the PEPFAR program. Therefore, many of the evaluation questions will require additional sources of data, analytical approaches, and methodologies. In the mixed methods approach described in this evaluation plan some limitations with readily obtained impact data may be overcome by using other proposed comparison methodologies, ancillary studies, key informant interviews, and site visits. These methods are described in more detail in the subsequent sections on evaluation methodologies and data sources. The type of methodology and analytical approach used to answer specific questions requested by Congress will differ depending on the rigor and feasibility of collecting existing data or the feasibility of gathering new information—as the committee intends to do during country visits and during interviews with OGAC staff, implementers, and other key stakeholders that will occur outside of country visits. This poses limitations on the evaluation approach and on the interpretation of the findings.

There are indicators that are reported centrally to OGAC across the entire PEPFAR program; however, these provide only limited answers to the evaluation charge. Although data from within PEPFAR that go beyond the centrally-reported indicators may be available, a preliminary scan of sources revealed that these data will have to come from disparate sources that are not currently catalogued or coordinated. These data sources, such as recommended indicators not reported to OGAC and data collected by the major USG implementing agencies and other implementation partners, are not managed through a process that allows for easy cataloguing of what is available from whom. Therefore, accessing the data to answer many of the evaluation questions will require a significant data-mapping and data-gathering effort that adds to the resource requirements of the evaluation. Requests from the IOM will also likely impose a burden of time and resources on staff at OGAC and other implementing agencies as well as on country teams and implementing partners; this introduces a dependence on the timely efforts of many different actors who, in many cases, are already overburdened.

Another possible source is data that are collected through other multilateral organizations and can be made available to the IOM. However, some of these data, as well as data from OGAC and implementing partners, are not already analyzed in a way that answers the questions posed by this evaluation in response to the congressional mandate. Therefore, to make full use of these data would require new analyses. In addition to questions requiring new analyses, some questions would require developing and using new data collection tools, which may or may not be feasible during the time period of the evaluation. Each of these approaches could enhance the quality of the evaluation, but each will also require a greater investment of resources than restricting the evaluation to existing data and analyses.

Another important limitation to note is that most of the additional data sources will not be PEPFAR-wide data or population data but will instead be country-specific, program-specific, or component-specific. When data are not collected systematically across all PEPFAR countries, this will limit the ability to generalize findings to the whole of the program. There is also considerable heterogeneity in the implementation of PEPFAR across different countries and programs, which limits the ability to generalize findings. However, country-specific, program-specific, or component-specific data can nonetheless be highly informative and, if interpreted with care, both commonalities and differences across countries can inform conclusions that contribute to an understanding of the performance and impact of PEPFAR as a whole.

In addition, it is important to note that, although substantial progress has been made in recent years to harmonize data collection, variability in the definitions of indicators and in the quality of available data will also be constraints to both the summary of findings and comparison of findings across countries, even when similar data are collected across multiple countries. This is especially true in some critical areas where consensus indicators have yet to be developed, such as health systems strengthening, integration of services, and country ownership.

Finally, there are also evaluation questions the committee will consider that will simply not be possible to answer in the forthcoming evaluation period. As part of the final evaluation report, questions of this kind may be discussed if they are found to be important for future ongoing evaluation, along with suggestions for how to develop the means to answer them.

## EVALUATION METHODOLOGIES

There are a number of alternative design and analysis techniques that could, in theory, be considered for inclusion in a mixed methods approach to the evaluation of the impact of the PEPFAR program. Each method has different requirements and each has its own strengths and weaknesses in terms of the types of evidence it brings to bear on a program evaluation. The range of methodological options in two main categories, comparison approaches and modeling, are described here as background information with a discussion of their relative advantages and disadvantages. The methods the committee found to have the potential to be feasible and relevant for this evaluation are then described in more detail, along with the potential sources of data for the evaluation.

### Comparison Approaches

One basic question is of paramount importance to decision makers in evaluating the effects of a program–what would have happened if the program had not been provided? This is often referred to as the "counter-factual." Answering this question requires an experimental design or analytical method that allows a comparison to be made over time between a group that receives the program and a group that does not. Ideally, these two groups would be similar enough to each other on key parameters that any difference in outcome would be attributable to the program itself rather than to other differences between the groups. There are a number of potential methodologies that could be considered to allow for these comparisons to be made.

In medical science, the randomized controlled trial is widely accepted as the "gold standard" in determining the effects of an intervention or in comparing one intervention to another (for example, to answer the question of whether one drug is better than another for treating an illness or preventing a medical outcome). The advantage of random assignment to intervention and comparison groups is that it should randomly distribute different characteristics between the two groups, thereby reducing the concern that pre-existing differences between the two groups, rather than the effect of the intervention, might account for the difference in outcomes. Randomization typically occurs at the level of the individual. However, in what is known as a cluster-randomized trial, randomization can also occur at a broader level, such as clinics, schools, or neighborhoods.

Randomized trials can provide useful evidence to evaluate components of a large-scale program, including not only interventions but also implementation questions or service delivery models. Indeed, some components provided within PEPFAR's activities have previously been evaluated for effectiveness using randomized trials, including ARV drugs and other pharmaceutical treatments as well as other interventions. For example, male circumcision as an intervention to reduce the transmission of HIV among young adults has been evaluated in three separate studies in three sub-Saharan countries (Auvert et al., 2005; Bailey et al., 2007; Gray et al., 2007). Behavioral interventions for HIV prevention have also been evaluated using randomized trials conducted in a variety of venues with a diversity of populations in sub-Saharan Africa (Cornman et al., 2008; Jemmott et al., in press; Jewkes et al., 2008; Kalichman et al., 2008; Stanton et al., 1998).

However, random assignment methodologies are not widely used to evaluate the effects of an entire large-scale, multi-component program because they require special conditions that cannot reasonably be met. In fact, it is difficult, and sometimes unethical, to have an appropriate control group that would comply with the parameters required in a randomized trial. First, when evaluating the delivery of proven interventions, control participants must be provided with the accepted standard of care because ethical considerations prevent withholding known effective treatments. This can lessen the difference between what the control and comparison groups receive, which can make it statistically difficult to detect an intervention effect, even with large and correspondingly expensive sample sizes. Second, it is not possible to "mask" the intervention for participants or to keep the control communities or participants "blinded" as to their experimental condition. In addition, random sampling is difficult to achieve in a large, widely implemented program, and the outcomes for any comparison group are likely to be affected by secular effects or by interventions or services provided through other programs. Finally, program interventions may also take a long time to have the desired effect, and it can be costly and impractical to maintain a trial for the required duration. Therefore, a randomized trial is often not considered feasible or appropriate for evaluating large-scale programs where the goal is to provide whole communities or entire districts with multiple, new services in the hopes of improving health outcomes.

There are alternative comparison methodologies that can be more feasible for evaluating large-scale programs, although challenges such as the timeframe of the trial and secular effects still apply. In a variation of a randomized evaluation approach, programs can be implemented in a phased rollout to different groups or areas over time, which can be randomly assigned. Although everyone eventually receives the intervention, phasing in the program in this way allows comparisons of outcome data in those that receive the program first against a control group made up of those not yet receiving the program (Hussey and Hughes, 2007). Conceivably, this design could be undertaken by countries that might, for example, choose to implement a new intervention or a new delivery mechanism in place of an established intervention district by district, allowing an evaluation of the impact on health outcomes.

Quasi-experimental studies also offer alternatives for assessing what would have happened in the absence of an intervention. These designs do not involve random assignment to intervention and control groups, but can allow comparisons between groups using a variety of approaches to control for differences between nonequivalent groups. One approach is to compare two groups or communities that are not randomized, but one is served by the program while the other is not. These can be planned comparison groups or can sometimes occur as "natural experiments" that serve as a variation on the phased rollout design described above. These occur when programmatic or policy changes are phased in. Data collected on outcomes in the groups or areas where the changes were implemented earlier versus later can produce informative evaluation data.

Ideally, these approaches would be designed to assess both the intervention and comparison groups before and after the program is delivered and then to analyze the "difference-in-differences" between the two groups. An alternative to this design is a "post-test" only comparison group. This is a comparison of similar groups in which the group that receives the intervention is measured before and after the intervention and is then compared at the "post-test" period to a similar group that had no exposure to the intervention. This approach can provide some valuable information to determine whether differences in outcomes can plausibly be associated with exposure to the intervention. In these comparisons, the concern in interpreting the results is that differences in outcomes may not be due to the program itself, but rather to other observed or unobserved differences between those who did and those who did not receive the intervention. To some extent, this concern can be addressed by matching the individuals or communities being compared on important characteristics that may affect the targeted outcomes, or by statistically accounting for any differences in these characteristics in the analysis of the data. However, this approach can be compromised by the possible influence of and inability to control for unobserved characteristics that may affect the outcomes.

When no appropriate comparison group is available, comparisons can also be made using before-after studies (also known as "pre-test/post-test"). These compare outcomes or indicators before a program was established to the same measures in the same group after the program was implemented. These studies are observational and not experimental in nature, but can allow the detection of significant change after the intervention is given. The disadvantage to this approach is the difficulty in controlling for other factors that may have coincided with the implementation of the program and may have caused or contributed to the observed changes. Data analysis of trends over time offers a similar method to inform an evaluation of the outcomes of a program across a range of metrics. If the trends in program inputs are associated with program activities on the ground and with later shifts in outcomes, it can be reasonable to conclude that the intervention program was plausibly important in changing the outcomes. However, this method requires that data collection be repeated reliably over time, which is often not the case for many data sources.

The challenge for evaluating a program such as PEPFAR, which is widely implemented at the national level across many countries, is that it can be very difficult to identify an appropriate comparison or control to use in the kinds of comparison approaches described previously. In addition, the ideal for comparison approaches would be to use a prospective design, in which data for both intervention and comparison groups are collected from the beginning of the evaluation. However, this is an evaluation that extends back in time to the implementation of a program well before the starting point of the evaluation. In addition, it is not feasible for the evaluation committee to mandate complex intervention and evaluation designs or new data collection in order to make prospective comparisons during the time period for this evaluation, although the committee will consider the outcomes of any such studies of PEPFAR program components if the findings are available by the end of the evaluation period. Instead, for most of the questions in this evaluation, comparisons can only be made retrospectively. This leads to the limitation that the evaluation committee will only have access to data that were already collected or are already being collected and as a result, the available data may be not be sufficient to answer all of the desired questions.

## Modeling

Methods employing mathematical and statistical models are another means of assessing health interventions and evaluating outcomes when an ideal experimental design with primary data collection is not practical or feasible. Analyses using these methods synthesize data from several sources to estimate the probable impact of different strategies. They can offer the advantages of analyzing different scenarios and projecting outcomes far into the future, both of which would be difficult to assess in a trial or in the field (Bertozzi, 2006; Garnett, 2002). However, models are dependent on the availability of accurate data sources, key input parameters, and epidemiological assumptions about disease transmission (Garnett, 2002). Many countries lack the necessary data to create a baseline from which future scenarios can be projected. Additionally, models rely heavily on published literature for impact parameters, which may overestimate the actual impact by focusing on high-quality, successful interventions (Forsythe et al., 2009). Therefore the reliability and utility of current modeling approaches need to be carefully assessed.

Countries, donors, and other global stakeholders use existing mathematical models to determine resource needs for HIV/AIDS programs and to make evidence-based decisions about future programming with the aim of achieving sustainability. These models require various inputs such as demographic, epidemiological, and financing data, and make various assumptions about the progression of disease. Thus, the validity of projections is conditional on the quality and completeness of existing data and the accuracy of the assumptions inherent to the model (Garnett, 2002). Until recently, PEPFAR focused on costing and modeling for ART (Holmes, 2009). However, PEPFAR has identified a continuum of costing and modeling activities and is transitioning from simply costing and forecasting ARV needs to modeling the cost of service delivery by measuring all inputs, including personnel, investments, and overheads. PEPFAR also plans to undertake comprehensive treatment costing and modeling of national program scenarios and is expanding costing exercises to include care and prevention. There are several models currently in use to estimate resources needs for interventions that the committee can consider as data sources, including the ART Cost Project (Levine, 2010), the HIV/AIDS Program Sustainability Analysis Tool (HAPSAT) (Dutta and Fleisher, 2008), and Spectrum Policy Modeling System (Constella Group LLC, 2008; Holmes, 2009).

In addition to modeling of costs and resource needs, mathematical modeling to estimate infections averted is of particular relevance because HIV incidence is difficult to measure directly. Three modeling approaches, coverage-based, behavior-based, and disease-modeling-based, have been proposed for estimating the number of HIV infections averted from intervention programs (Heaton et al., 2008). The coverage-based approach relies on an estimate of the efficacy of the intervention on incident HIV infection. By incorporating coverage information associated with the intervention (e.g. numbers of persons receiving the intervention), estimates are produced through models of the number of infections averted. Two critical inputs (the coverage and the relative risk) are important sources of uncertainty with this approach (Heaton et al., 2008). A second approach, the behavior-based approach, relies on a model that describes how HIV infection is mediated by behavior. Two critical inputs to this approach are evidence of the effects of behavior change on incident HIV infection and the change in prevalence of the high-risk behaviors resulting from the intervention. A key limitation of this method is the lack of reliable behavioral data in many developing countries. The third approach, the disease modeling approach, is based on a comparison of observed HIV incidence trends with the expected or baseline HIV incidence trends. However, few countries have been able to collect true population-level incidence data and there have been difficulties with measuring incidence using measures such as BED immunoassays[12] (Hallett et al., 2009; Murphy and Parry, 2008). It has also been suggested that, as an alternative, HIV prevalence trends among young persons (ages 15–24 years) can be assessed as an approximation of incidence (UNAIDS and WHO, 2009). Likewise, some have found that serial cross-sectional prevalence data may be used to estimate general-population incidence by age (Hallett et al., 2008). Indirect strategies for estimating HIV incidence include models, such as the Estimation and Projection Package and the Spectrum software, developed at UNAIDS, that have been used by some researchers to predict HIV prevalence. Comparisons of the observed trends with the modeled or expected trends have been used to estimate infections averted.

PEPFAR's estimates of the number of infections averted in partner countries are produced by the U.S. Census Bureau (PEPFAR, 2010a). The Census Bureau model (known as, RUPHIVAIDS) follows a disease-modeling approach in which expected or baseline HIV incidence estimates are developed with data prior to 2005 and compared to re-estimated trends in HIV incidence from new surveillance data available after 2004. The difference in the number of new infections, based on this comparison approach, is used as the number of infections averted. The model incorporates estimates of HIV prevalence from the Estimation and Projection Package to project HIV incidence and applies various assumptions in relation to sex distribution of HIV infection, sex ratios of new infections, rate of mother-to-child transmission, and disease progression as recommended by the UNAIDS Reference Group on Estimates, Modelling and Projections (U.S. Census Bureau, 2009).

Modeling of infections averted can also be used to specifically measure the impact of PMTCT on vertical (mother-to-child) transmission of HIV. For example, both HAPSAT and the Spectrum Suite can be used to project the number of infections averted through ART, ARV prophylaxis, and improved breastfeeding techniques (Constella Group LLC, 2008; Dutta and Fleisher, 2008). These estimates are limited by the quality and availability of data regarding the percent of women with access to PMTCT that agree to be tested, the percent of women found to be HIV-positive that accept ARV prophylaxis and/or substitute feeding, and the percent reduction in the rate of mother-to-child transmission with prophylactic treatment and/or substitute feeding (Resch et al., 2009, UNAIDS, 2009b).

It will not be feasible for the evaluation committee to conduct new mathematical modeling. However, the committee will consider the strengths and weaknesses of existing modeling efforts, such as those described, and will assess the reliability of the estimates they provide in the two areas that are relevant to PEPFAR: (1) the cost of HIV/AIDS interventions and the resources necessary to scale up and maintain programs and (2) infections averted. Where deemed appropriate, these estimates will be used as a source of data for the committee's assessment of PEPFAR's outcomes and impact.

---

[12] The BED-CEIA (HIV-1 subtype B, CRF_01AE, and subtype D–Capture Enzyme Immunoassay) is a commercially available product designed specifically for the purpose of indentifying HIV-1 infections that were recently acquired—using the three specific peptides to cover much of the extent of antigenic diversity to overcome some of the subtype differences associated with the "detuned" assays (Murphy and Parry, 2008).

**Application of Methodologies in the PEPFAR Evaluation**

Given these methodological design considerations, the evaluation will employ a mix of quantitative and qualitative methods, including trend analysis and retrospective comparison approaches using quantitative analysis of key indicators, document review, mapping of resources, policy analysis, benchmarking of outputs and outcomes against stated goals, site visits, and primary data collection through structured interviews and town hall meetings with key informants. Where feasible, methods will be applied and data will be gathered at the level of the whole of the program or for all of the PEPFAR partner countries. However, in order to not limit all findings to the constraints on consistent data availability across the whole of the program and all of the countries, the committee will also identify countries, programmatic areas, or intervention components implemented within PEPFAR for which a methodology cannot feasibly be applied consistently for all PEPFAR countries or data may not be available for all countries, but where sufficient data can be gathered to allow in-depth studies to assess effects, including outcomes and impact. These in-depth studies may be specific to individual PEPFAR countries or, in some instances, a multi-country analysis may be feasible. For example, some prevention and treatment activities have been subject to multiple evaluations that have been conducted on a smaller scale than the whole of PEPFAR, but when reviewed in depth will nonetheless serve to inform the committee's overall findings.

By applying this mix of methods and layers of investigation and analysis using a range of available primary and secondary data sources (see Boxes 2a–d in the section that follows), the committee will arrive at findings that can be triangulated to draw conclusions about the performance and impact of PEPFAR even when any one data source is not sufficient or any one methodological approach is not feasible.

*PEPFAR Country Studies*

Given the limitations on data that can be gathered at the level of the whole of the program, a major area of focus for the evaluation will be country studies. A country-by-country approach offers a potentially rich source of evaluation data. Country studies will be used by the evaluation committee to assess progress of the program at the country level against targets set in national AIDS strategies and in the PEPFAR COP. Country studies are also an opportunity to conduct time-series and trend analyses that compare outcomes before and after PEPFAR programs were implemented or before and after changes in PEPFAR programs were introduced within a country. In addition, although there will be limits to aggregating or generalizing country-specific findings due to the heterogeneity across PEPFAR countries, country-by-country assessments can, if interpreted carefully, contribute to conclusions about the performance and impact of PEPFAR as a whole. Country studies will also provide the necessary data collection to make the cross-country comparisons described later. The main component of these country studies will be country data sets that will be compiled for each of the current PEPFAR partner countries using key indicators gathered from OGAC and other available data sources as well as document review (see Boxes 2a–d).

To the extent possible, local experts, governments, organizations, and implementing partners at the country level will be engaged in the evaluation process. The committee will solicit their assistance in determining the availability and quality of country-specific and program-specific data sources and will seek to collect data, including data from national health information systems, as well as data analyses developed and conducted by local experts. The planning committee strongly endorses the principle of engaging country-level partners and considers this a potentially important component of the evaluation, which would also be consistent with PEPFAR's goals to strengthen country capacity to monitor as well as manage the AIDS epidemic (OGAC, 2009g). However, the committee also recognizes that additional requests for data and analysis can place a significant burden on local partners that is not accounted for in current planning or budgeting. Therefore, the committee will seek to maximize engagement within the bounds of what will realistically be feasible. Pilot country visits during the operational planning phase will provide an opportunity to explore and assess the feasibility of engaging country experts in the evaluation process.

**Country data sets** The committee will identify and request relevant documents and other data sources to build country data sets for each country and to perform content analysis. These will include key indicators from PEPFAR and other multilateral agencies, as well as national M&E systems, data extracted from country team and national planning and reporting documents, and available data from the published literature, grey literature, and prior evaluations. Sources of data that will inform these country data sets are listed in more detail in Boxes 2a–d. In addition to informing data sets across all countries, this document review will help the committee identify countries and programmatic areas for in-depth studies.

**Country timelines** A country timeline will be developed for each of PEPFAR's current partner countries to provide an overview for the past 12 years of major events related to the epidemic and HIV/AIDS programs and to map the timing of the availability of key data sources (see Appendix E for example timelines). These country timelines will serve as a multi-purpose evaluation tool. First, they will inform the analysis and interpretation of trends and longitudinal data for some of the outcome and impact indicators. For example, they will illustrate which countries have surveillance data that have been repeated before and after the implementation of PEPFAR and which countries have had policy changes or changes to their national health systems since PEPFAR activities began. In addition, they will map the presence and timing of other contextual factors that may affect the interpretation of PEPFAR's contribution to health impact. Lastly they will provide a snapshot of the data available at the country level which can be used to select and design different analyses (e.g., comparison studies) and in-depth studies (e.g., country visits).

The main types of information that will be gathered to build the country timelines are PEPFAR activities, the major activities and investments of other donors, and country- and global-level policy information that would be expected to have an impact on the countries' response to the HIV epidemic. This will be overlaid with information on recent and past data availability as well as new data anticipated to become available during the evaluation timeframe, especially population-based surveys and other HIV-related surveillance data. The information will be drawn from a number of sources, concurrent with the process for country data sets described above (see Boxes 2a–d). These sources will include published literature and PEPFAR-related documents from OGAC, U.S. agencies, and other PEPFAR implementing partners, as well as country-specific global stakeholder reports and other external evaluations. Additionally, global health or health policy media outlets will be used as a source of information on events related to the HIV/AIDS epidemic in the each country.

**Country visits** While some in-depth studies will be conducted through document review, the evaluation committee will also visit select countries for in-depth studies. These country visits will serve a number of goals. A primary purpose of the country visits will be to obtain qualitative data, including semi-structured interviews with key informants and observational data. This is particularly critical for the committee to collect information on process questions related to the implementation of PEPFAR programs, including barriers to implementation, harmonization with national plans, and indirect or unintended effects as observed by local authorities and implementing partners. A main focus will be to gather information on whether the program is implemented according to PEPFAR guidance, with an emphasis on the new PEPFAR II Five-Year Strategic Plan for transitioning to a sustainable response. This will include an assessment of progress toward goals such as country ownership, capacity building, health systems strengthening, resources, transparency and accountability, and other program characteristics deemed essential for a sustainable response. Country visits can also inform the committee's assessment of progress toward other program targets for which limited quantitative data may be available, such as implementation of strategies to address gender issues and to reach vulnerable populations. These questions will not be readily addressed through existing data sources and are dependent on observations of the program made in context.

The information gathered from these country visits will also inform the interpretation of quantitative data by providing context for baseline country characteristics and trends in the epidemic, for the heterogeneity of the implementation of PEPFAR across countries, and for assessments of data quality. In some cases, the country visits will also allow the committee to collect additional locally-available quantitative data. Additionally, the country visits are an opportunity to obtain country-specific information on funding flows, on the costs of interventions, and on efforts and outcomes in PEPFAR's programmatic areas.

*Selection of countries for country visits* Due to limited resources and time, it will not be feasible to conduct country visits to all of the current PEPFAR countries. Instead, the committee will use purposive sampling to select a subset of countries that represent a diverse range on a number of key characteristics. These will include but will not be limited to: (1) the types of interventions and activities implemented with PEPFAR funding, (2) the operational infrastructure (especially the distribution pattern of funding), (3) the size of country, (4) the size of financial inputs from PEPFAR and other sources, (5) the length of time PEPFAR programs have been in place, (6) epidemic trends and epidemic type (concentrated versus generalized), and (7) country income level. The data to be collected will be further defined based on the country case study framework and key evaluation questions that are best addressed during a country site visit.

*Country visit process and standardization* The following describes the strategy that will be used for data collection and standardization for country visits. The operational planning phase will include pilot testing and refining of these methods. As an independent and neutral third party, the IOM country visit teams are expected to be reasonably able to elicit candid information from key informants. To help encourage this candor, the committee will not attribute comments, examples, or findings to specific informants without express permission.

1. Preparation for country visits:
   - Develop the country visit case study framework and data analysis plan to ensure consistency in methodology across countries to allow for comparisons linked to key evaluation questions

- Review country-specific background information to generate hypotheses and determine questions to be probed in-country
  - Review of PEPFAR and national indicator data
  - Document review and preparation of country timelines (described previously)
- Develop interview questions for different categories of interviewees (i.e., PEPFAR agency, PEPFAR implementer, PEPFAR beneficiary; country partner, international partner)
- Develop framework and criteria for observational data collection
- Develop and prepare a country visit qualitative data collection toolkit for use by IOM evaluation teams on country visits
- Train committee members and staff on data collection tools and data reporting methods
- Agree on a date for the country visit, identify interviewees for each country, and schedule interview and site visit appointments

2. Process for country visits (see Appendix F for details):
   - Time frame: January through August 2011
   - Duration: 7–14 days (depending on size of country, size of program, and what evaluation questions are relevant for each country study)
   - Number of countries: 12–15
   - Investigation teams: 3 IOM committee members, 2 IOM staff, and consultants and contractors as needed
   - Stakeholders to interview:
     - PEPFAR: U.S. Ambassador, CDC, USAID, PEPFAR implementing partners, program beneficiaries
     - Partner country stakeholders: National AIDS Commission; Ministries of Health, Finance, and other relevant ministries; civil society representatives; other relevant local stakeholders
     - Country-level representatives of other external programs: UNAIDS, other United Nations agencies, Global Fund Country Coordinating Mechanism members, Global Fund recipients, World Bank, other bilateral donors

3. Post country site visit follow-up activities:
   - Country visit write up (within 4 weeks after visit)
   - On-going analyses of quantitative and qualitative data

## Comparisons Among Countries Within PEPFAR

In addition to country-by-country studies, the evaluation committee will consider conducting comparisons among countries within PEPFAR after weighing the feasibility of this approach based on data mapping during the operational planning period. The goal of this comparison approach would be to determine if changes in key indicators in a PEPFAR country are associated with variables such as the timing of the introduction of PEPFAR into that country; the scale of the PEPFAR presence in that country (as measured, for example, by the extent of funding and activities); or the operational infrastructure (including, for example, how PEPFAR funding is distributed among implementing partners or the extent to which PEPFAR activities are parallel to or integrated within public sector health services).

One approach to implementing such an analysis would begin by assembling a database on changes in key indicators over time in each PEPFAR country. The dependent variables would be the relative or percentage changes in key indicators over defined time intervals. Adjusted analyses could then be performed that correlate those changes in key indicators with explanatory variables such as the duration of time PEPFAR had been present in the country, the cumulative PEPFAR investment in the country up to that point in time, and differing PEPFAR implementation strategies. The committee recognizes that there are critical differences among PEPFAR countries with respect to demographics, social and economic factors, and the epidemiology of the epidemic that must be taken into account in these analyses. Accordingly, adjusted analyses must be performed that carefully consider and account for such confounding factors. To determine the feasibility of this approach, the committee will assemble a database of country level variables thought to be related to the propagation of the epidemic and consider their use in adjusted analyses of comparisons among PEPFAR countries. A major limitation of this approach is uncertainties in some of the key benchmark indicators including HIV prevalence and HIV-related deaths. The committee also recognizes the limitations of these analyses for inferring causation based on associations.

An additional approach for comparison analyses that the committee will consider will be to compare sub-units within PEPFAR countries that receive different levels of PEPFAR investment or where different types of PEPFAR activities have been implemented. This alternative may allow for comparisons among groups that are more similar in baseline characteristics and available data, although there may still be limitations due to regional differences in demographics, social and economic factors, the epidemiology of the epidemic, and availability of the appropriate data.

*Comparisons Between PEPFAR and Non-PEPFAR Countries*

Another approach to the evaluation of PEPFAR that will be considered for the evaluation is based on comparisons of PEPFAR to non-PEPFAR countries with respect to key indicators.[13] The operational planning for the evaluation will allow time to gather the data necessary to fully review the utility of this approach in light of the limitations described below. The evaluation committee will assess the strength of the evidence about the effectiveness of PEPFAR that can be gleaned from comparisons of PEPFAR to non-PEPFAR countries and will only conduct these comparisons if deemed appropriate.

The committee recognizes that PEPFAR focus countries were not chosen randomly. Therefore, there are important differences between PEPFAR focus countries and non-PEPFAR countries that must be accounted for if a comparison approach is to be valid. These differences relate to economic, political, and health factors; population sizes; the stage of the epidemic; and

---

[13] A comparison of 12 PEPFAR focus countries with generalized epidemics in Africa to 29 control countries was recently published (Bendavid and Bhattacharya, 2009). This correlational analysis, using UNAIDS data as the source for outcomes indicators, showed a significantly more rapid decrease in the rate of deaths due to HIV/AIDS in the PEPFAR focus countries than in non-PEPFAR countries during the period of PEPFAR activities between 2004 and 2007. The authors noted the difficulties of generalizing the findings to other countries and other time periods because of the non-random sampling of the comparison groups. There were baseline differences between the intervention and control groups in variables such as population, adult HIV prevalence, gross domestic product, aid targeted to HIV/AIDS from other donor sources, and World Bank indicators of governance. The authors reported that adjusted analyses to account for these variables did not change the significance or direction of the reported findings, which were the results of unadjusted analyses.

available infrastructure and capacity prior to the introduction of PEPFAR. In addition, many countries where PEPFAR has not been implemented may have implemented similar interventions to achieve the same objective through programs with support from other external or national funding sources. When this is the case, comparisons cannot evaluate the presence or absence of the intervention activities supported by PEPFAR per se, but rather the implementation and delivery strategy used by PEPFAR. As a result, the approach of comparing PEPFAR to non-PEPFAR countries would require special care in implementation, analysis, and interpretation.

For this kind of comparison approach to be useful for this evaluation, it would be critical to identify control countries that can be suitably compared to PEPFAR countries. The control counties would be selected from the same geographic regions as the PEPFAR countries (e.g., sub-Saharan Africa, Asia, the Russian Federation or Eurasia, and the Caribbean). The evaluation committee's work would begin by assembling a database of baseline country-level variables in both PEPFAR and non-PEPFAR countries that might relate to the course of the epidemic. The committee will also document investments in HIV activities from country governments and external donors. The validity of using this comparison approach to draw reliable inferences about the effects of PEPFAR will depend on whether the analyses can be adequately adjusted to make fair comparisons between PEPFAR and the candidate non-PEPFAR control countries. Adjusted analyses that statistically control for differences will be considered. The dependent variables in the adjusted analyses will be the relative or percentage changes in key indicators before and after introduction of PEPFAR. The before-after percentage changes in PEPFAR countries will be compared to non-PEPFAR countries, adjusting for differences in baseline variables and taking into account HIV activities supported from other sources. As with the comparisons among countries within PEPFAR, a major limitation is that there are important uncertainties in some of the key benchmark indicators used as the dependent variables, such as HIV prevalence and numbers of HIV-related deaths. In addition, there are a number of measures of interest for this evaluation for which data are not collected across PEPFAR and non-PEPFAR countries, which would limit the scope of this approach in addressing many of the evaluation questions drawn from the statement of task.

## DATA SOURCES AND ANALYSIS

The extent to which the goals of this evaluation can be met depends on the availability of relevant and timely data. As described previously, most evaluation questions will require the evaluation committee to draw on data that go beyond the indicators that are reported centrally to OGAC. These data will have to come from a range of disparate sources. The availability of this data will partly depend on the feasibility of access within the timeframe of the evaluation. There will also be challenges of sampling and interpretation due to heterogeneous data sources with different data collection systems and criteria, as well as the potential for reporting bias in the responses to data requests from the committee. The approach for collecting and assessing data that could be used for the evaluation is described here and in the subsequent section on the workplan for the evaluation.

### Mapping of Data Sources

The time and resources available for the planning phase did not allow for a complete mapping of all currently available and anticipated data sources in time for this report. In the operational planning period the IOM staff, under the guidance of the planning committee, will continue an extensive data-mapping effort, expanding on the preliminary scan of data sources conducted during this strategic planning phase. The mapping will occur through document review, informant interviews, information obtained from domestic and international data requests, and qualitative methods used during three pilot country visits. The timing of this evaluation, with a final report to be delivered in 2012, dictates that the committee will be considering only data that are or will become available to the committee through 2011.

This mapping will determine what data are available for each of the PEPFAR countries, providing the evaluation committee with a data matrix similar to the template that can be found in Appendix G. Some of these data sources will also be mapped for non-PEPFAR countries to inform the feasibility of the comparison approaches described earlier—these approaches would rely on the availability of data from these countries, and on the willingness and capacity of stakeholders in non-PEPFAR countries to participate in country visits and other data-gathering requests. This mapping of available data will also include an assessment of the feasibility of collecting data from each source, taking into consideration the burden that additional data requests would place on each source's resources and staff time. In addition, this data mapping will assess whether data from each source would require new data analysis in order to answer the evaluation questions posed by the committee.

The categories and some examples of available data sources that will be mapped and, if available, used for the evaluation are listed in Boxes 2a–d. These include central USG data sources, data from multilateral organizations, country-level data from both PEPFAR and other sources, and data from additional sources, which may be from single countries or multiple countries. The applicability of specific data sources to address illustrative evaluation questions in some specific programmatic areas will be discussed in the subsequent sections of this report.

**BOX 2a**
**Central U.S. Government Data Sources**

**Office of the U.S. Global AIDS Coordinator (OGAC) Reports and Planning/Guidance Documents:** OGAC periodically releases reports of its activities as well as programmatic, policy, and reporting guidance for field programs. Most of the reports are requested by Congress or required under federal regulations. Guidance for field programs includes both formal guidance documents and other communications from headquarters to implementing partners and country teams.

- 5-year strategic plans
- Country Operational Plan guidance
- PEPFAR indicators reference guide (including the Next Generation Indicators Reference Guide)
- Programmatic guidance
- Partnership Frameworks and Partnership Framework Implementation Plans Guidance
- Public health evaluation guidance
- Reporting guidance for the annual program results (APRs)/semi-annual progress results (SPRs)
- PEPFAR annual reports and other reports to Congress
- PEPFAR operational plans
- Obligation and outlay reports
- PEPFAR State of the Program Area
- News to the Field

**Data Reported to OGAC through the Country Operational Plan Reporting System (COPRS II):** As part of PEPFAR's monitoring and evaluation (M&E) of activities, countries are required to report program data through COPRS II. Countries submit two reports to OGAC annually (APRs and SAPRs), which include data from the essential and reported PEPFAR indicators* collected from implementing partners on all technical areas.

**Congressional Appropriations Bills and Conference Reports:** The U.S. House of Representatives and U.S. Senate Committees on Appropriations and their appropriate subcommittees have the broad responsibility over the discretionary budget for global HIV/AIDS bilateral funding and the U.S. government funding for multilateral organizations such as the Global Fund to Fight AIDS, Tuberculosis and Malaria.

**Office of Management and Budget (OMB):** OMB Circulars are instructions or information issued by OMB to federal agencies. These are expected to have a continuing effect of 2 years or more. PEPFAR funding for HIV/AIDS is subjected to OMB Circulars.

**PEPFAR Implementing Agencies Data:** Program monitoring, evaluation, and research data as well as other relevant information over which these agency have oversight (e.g., principally the Office of HIV/AIDS within the Global Health Bureau at the United States Agency for International Development [USAID] and the Global AIDS Program at the U.S. Centers for Disease Control and Prevention).

**PEPFAR External Evaluations:** Reports of evaluations of PEPFAR conducted by other U.S. government agencies, including the Government Accountability Office. Congressional Research Service, OMB, and the Offices of the Inspector General for the Department of State, USAID, and the Department of Health and Human Services. These include reports on topics such as program management and implementation, coordination, funding allocations and oversight, technical assistance, harmonization, and program efficiency and effectiveness.[a]

* PEPFAR guidance classifies indicators in three ways: by degree of importance and aggregation level (i.e., essential and reported to headquarters, essential and not reported to headquarter, or recommended indicators), by reporting level (i.e., direct program or national indicators), and by standard M&E classification (i.e., output, outcome, or impact indicators).

SOURCE: Compiled from U.S. Government publicly available information and PEPFAR's website (www.pepfar.gov).
[a]For example: CRS (2005,2007, 2008a, 2008b, 2009); DoS OIG (2008, 2009); GAO (2004, 2005, 2006, 2008, 2009).

**BOX 2b**
**Multilateral Donor and Other International Data Sources**

Multilateral donors and international organizations play an active role in implementing global commitments on HIV/AIDS and supporting these through funding and technical assistance. Data available from multilateral donors and international organizations are reported by national governments, which are generally required to report on the progress of externally supported HIV/AIDS programs. The following are examples of these types of sources of data:

**Joint United Nations Programme on HIV/AIDS (UNAIDS)**
- Global HIV statistics and other estimates (e.g., "Report on the Global AIDS Epidemic" and "AIDS Epidemic Update" reports)
- Frameworks and Indexes (e.g., National Composite Policy Index and Stigma Index)
- National AIDS spending assessments
- United Nations General Assembly Special Session on HIV and AIDS country progress reports
- Project and indicator data collected, analyzed, and reported through the Country Response Information System or the Indicator Registry

**United Nations Children's Fund (UNICEF)**
- HIV Statistics and other socio-economic statistics affecting child well-being (i.e., "State of the World's Children" annual reports)
- Frameworks (e.g., Five-year global campaign on children and AIDS)
- Publications (e.g., the "Children and AIDS Stocktaking Reports")
- Technical and policy documents
- Review of status of programs (addressing focus areas: preventing mother-to-child transmission of HIV; providing pediatric treatment; preventing infection among adolescents and young people; protecting and supporting children affected by HIV and AIDS)

**World Health Organization (WHO)**
- Data and statistics (e.g., data on testing and counselling, mother-to-child transmission of HIV, antiretroviral therapy, and pediatric HIV)
- National Health Accounts
- Country-specific antiretroviral drug costs
- HIV drug resistance monitoring reports and literature
- WHO normative guidance and publications
- The International Health Regulations 2005

**The Global Fund to Fight AIDS, Tuberculosis and Malaria (Global Fund)**
- National Health Accounts
- Progress reports including technical support grants from PEPFAR
- Key performance indicators
- Global Fund five-year evaluation: Study area 3 report[a]
- Global Fund evaluation country case studies

**The World Bank**
- Public expenditure reviews
- Project documents
- Analytic work/research
- Health and HIV/AIDS project evaluations
- Evaluation of HIV/AIDS support Bank-wide[b]
- Country assistance evaluations

**Organisation for Economic Co-operation and Development (OECD)**
- HIV-related funding data
- Country surveys
- Evaluation studies

**Other Multilateral or International Data Sources:**
- aids2031 reports and working papers
- Committee on the Rights of the Child, States reports
- Millennium Development Goals reports
- UNITAID reports
- European HIV/AIDS Funders Group
- Interagency Group for Mortality Estimation
- Funders Concerned about AIDS

SOURCE: Compiled from the Global Fund, OECD, UNAIDS, UNICEF, WHO, and World Bank publicly available information and personal communications with individuals at these organizations.
[a]TERG (2009).
[b]For example: IEG World Bank (2009) and World Bank (2007).

**BOX 2c**
**Country Data Sources**

**PEPFAR Country Sources:** Program data and other information generated at the country level.
- Country operational plan (fiscal years 2004–2011)
- Partnership framework and implementation plan
- Prime and sub-prime partner reports
- OGAC indicators not centrally reported*
- HIV Programs costing data
- Other communications among country teams and implementing partners

**National Policy Documents and other National AIDS Response Information:** Relevant national policy documents, strategies, and plans of action supporting PEPFAR activities and/or beneficiaries of PEPFAR-funded activities.

- National AIDS Coordinating Authority's strategy and framework
- Agencies or departments policy documents and plans (e.g., Ministries of Health, Finance)
- Country harmonization and alignment tool surveys

**National Health Information Systems:** National health information systems play an important role in ensuring that reliable and timely health information is available for operational and strategic decision making about HIV/AIDS country programs.
- Census data
- Civil registration and vital statistics
- Ministries of Health and Finance data
- Health services records
- Population surveys (e.g., Multiple Indicator Cluster Survey, Demographic and Health Survey, AIDS Indicator Survey, Behavioral Surveillance Survey, and Biologic and Behavioral Surveillance Survey)
- Antenatal care surveillance data
- Facility surveys (e.g., Service Provision Assessment and Service Availability Mapping)

*Additional essential/not reported to headquarters and recommended indicators beyond the 25 essential indicators reported to headquarters collected at the country and partner level.

SOURCE: Compiled from publicly available information and personal communications.

---

**BOX 2d**
**Other Data Sources (Single or Multi-Country)**

**Public Health Evaluations:** Concept papers, protocols, and/or progress reports for each approved PEPFAR public health evaluation (PHE). PHEs are investigator-initiated studies intended to guide the PEPFAR program and future policy development, to provide evidence to the HIV/AIDS community on programs that work, and to identify gaps in knowledge that can be filled with timely program evaluation and research.

**Published Literature:** Peer-reviewed journal articles, grey literature, and other reports relevant to PEPFAR's activities. These will address country-specific or program-specific studies as well as technical areas such as operations research of HIV programs, prevention of mother-to-child transmission, sexual prevention, blood safety, injection safety, intravenous and non-intravenous drug use, male circumcision, adult and pediatric care and treatment, tuberculosis and HIV co-infection, counseling and testing, health systems strengthening, gender-related HIV issues.

**Existing Modeling Data Sources for Costing:** PEPFAR works with countries in estimating resources needs for interventions. At the country-level, PEPFAR uses several models including the ART Cost Project, HIV/AIDS Program Sustainability Analysis Tool, and Spectrum Policy Modeling System.

**Existing Modeling Data Sources for HIV Infections Averted:** Since the numbers of HIV infections averted due to the implementation of a specific intervention(s) cannot be measured directly, modeling approaches provide a proxy to measure impact (e.g., models that estimate the efficacy of the intervention on incident HIV infection, models that describe how HIV infections are mediated by behavior, and models that compare incidence trends with the expected or baseline HIV incidence trends).

SOURCE: Compiled from publicly available information and personal communications.

---

**Analysis and Interpretation of Data**

The evaluation committee will guide the implementation of the evaluation and data analysis, interpret the data, and deliberate to come to consensus on the findings, conclusions, and recommendations. Primary data and secondary data that require additional analysis will be analyzed, using appropriate statistical methodologies, by the members of the evaluation committee and, with the committee's guidance, by the study staff team, which will be augmented for the implementation of the evaluation with additional staff trained in statistical analysis and data management. In addition, the committee will use specific subcontractor services for some areas where there is specialized knowledge needed with a substantial time commitment above what the volunteer committee members can provide. For example, expert consultation will contribute to the design of the tools and methods for qualitative data collection and to oversight of the analysis of primary qualitative data collected during country visits, other structured interviews, and other qualitative methods. Expert consultation will also be used to advise and assist in designing and supervising appropriate data requests and quantitative/qualitative analysis of secondary data. The committee will oversee all analyses performed by subcontractors to ensure validity and rigor as well as integration with the overall evaluation methodology.

The committee, staff, and consultants will take steps to quantify the quality and completeness of the data used for the evaluation. For the primary data collected by the committee, the methods used to assure the quality of the data will be described in full in the final report. When existing data analyses are used, the committee will review and assess the methodology and quality of the data in the original analyses. When secondary data are requested and used for new analyses conducted by the committee, a request will also be made for a description of the data management plan, and the committee will assess the procedures in place to assure the quality of the data, including, whenever possible, parameters such as reporting rates, sampling frame, and data completeness. This information will allow the evaluation committee to assess possible reporting bias and data quality and take these factors into account to inform the evaluation committee's interpretation of the data based on the likely reliability and quality. In its final report, the committee will include an accounting of data requests as well as a summary and analysis of the data quality and completeness. This will include the number of data requests made and the extent to which these requests were completed as requested. For data requests within PEPFAR, this will also afford the committee an opportunity to assess the completeness and validity of data as a metric of program progress toward sufficient data collection capacity for M&E, a critical component of sustainability. Although the assessment of data requests and data quality will be reported in the aggregate, data request outcomes will not be linked in the report to the specific organizations that receive data requests to avoid inhibiting the reporting of data.

## WORKPLAN

### Operational Planning Phase

As the culmination of the planning phase for this study, a transitional operational planning period will take place between the delivery of this report and the implementation of the evaluation itself. As described previously, the operational planning activities were intentionally structured and approved by Congress and OGAC as part of an ongoing planning phase, after delivery of the report, so that work on the evaluation could continue uninterrupted and so that the evaluation committee would not be starting de novo with respect to data availability and cataloguing, pilot-testing of instruments and methods, and development of relationships with relevant stakeholders. The results of these operational planning activities will be detailed in staff-authored planning documents for the evaluation committee as part of their background information and preparation to implement the evaluation.

Activities in this period will be carried out by IOM staff and planning committee members and will be designed to further develop and refine the plan described here and to inform the implementation of the evaluation. The operational planning will focus on data mapping (sources and availability of relevant data); mapping of methods and data sources, including key indicators, to the mandated tasks and illustrative questions in order to refine and prioritize key evaluation questions and identify key indicators; developing procedures for data requests; initiating data requests; designing and initiating data quality review methods for data received; refining and testing country visit selection criteria; preparing country timelines and other background materials for PEPFAR countries, and developing country study frameworks and methods for country visits. Some initial structured interviews with key informants will also take place during the operational planning period, and a final operational planning task will be continued relationship-building with relevant stakeholders such as contacts in PEPFAR countries and at implementing partner organizations.

Initial discussions with OGAC staff about data availability and the preliminary data scan conducted during this planning phase revealed that much of the data that the committee will need are not available through the headquarters level. In addition, the committee learned that implementing partners, agencies, and countries do not necessarily have to share a lot of their available data with OGAC. In light of this, OGAC agreed to partner with the IOM to help facilitate, to the extent they are able, access to these data by making introductions to field, headquarters, and agency staff and by disseminating information about the purpose of the evaluation. An initial introduction was sent in a News-to-the-Field posting from OGAC on June 4, 2010, which explained the mandate for the study, the progress of the planning committee as of the posting date, the proposed data-mapping activities and pilot country visits during the operational planning phase, and that the IOM data requests, country visits, site visits, and interview would be entirely independent of the relationship of implementing partners and other country-level stakeholders with OGAC and other USG implementing agencies. It also assured that the evaluation is not a financial audit or evaluation of specific programs; that findings, examples, and comments would not be attributed without expressed permission; and that participation in the evaluation is voluntary.[14]

Operational planning activities will also include the use of a qualitative research and evaluation consultant. This consultant will help to develop and refine data collection instruments and processes for country visits, in-depth studies, and other qualitative data collection; to determine what design issues, options, and qualitative methods beyond interviewing might be appropriate and feasible (e.g., content/thematic, statistical, or combination analyses; systematic triangulation; focus groups; direct observations for contextual information; town halls; photovoice); to plan logistics for field work; to test illustrative questions for refinement; to make determinations about the balance of breadth versus depth within the design options and data collection instruments; to develop audit trails to assure rigor of the fieldwork; and to train IOM staff in qualitative methods and the use of qualitative analytical software. In addition, pilot testing and refinement of field research methods and data collection instruments, with the qualitative consultant, will occur during visits to three PEPFAR countries, one bilaterally- and two multilaterally-funded.

## Implementation Phase

The evaluation committee will produce one consensus report with its findings and recommendations. This report is targeted for delivery to Congress by Fall of 2012. The overall time line for the evaluation will be approximately 24 months. The first 18 months will be data collection and analysis, building on the activities of the operational planning phase. This will also include consultation with relevant domestic and international stakeholders, implementing partners, and others with relevant expertise. The remaining six months will include final data analysis and interpretation of findings, determination of conclusions and recommendations by consensus among the committee members, finalization of the committee's report, an

---

[14] Personal communication from OGAC, June 4, 2010.

institutionally-overseen peer-report review, report production, and briefings for the sponsor as requested.

Over the course of the evaluation, the full committee will meet at least four times in person, with participation of the subcontractors and consultants. Additional virtual meetings will be conducted as needed using videoconferencing, teleconferencing, and web-based conferencing tools. In addition, working groups within the committee focused on specific content areas will hold in-person and virtual meetings, as needed, for ongoing deliberations as well as data analysis and interpretation. These committee activities will be augmented by ongoing communications, by telephone and electronic mail among the committee members, staff, and subcontractors and consultants.

A summary schematic of the proposed work plan and timeline for the evaluation can be found in Appendix F. Adjustments may be needed to the timeline and work plan due to any delay in the start time of the evaluation phase or to uncontrollable external shocks such as man-made or natural disasters (e.g., Haitian earthquake), political instability that could jeopardize the safety of members in countries that are identified for committee visits, or unforeseen scheduling problems for traveling (e.g., the Icelandic volcano eruption in 2010).

# PART III

# Illustrative Evaluation Details for Assessment of PEPFAR's Performance and Impact

The IOM was mandated by Congress in the Lantos–Hyde Act of 2008 to conduct a study that includes an assessment of the performance of U.S.-assisted global HIV/AIDS programs and an evaluation of the impact on health of prevention, treatment, and care efforts that are supported by U.S. funding. Part of the charge to the planning committee in developing a plan for this evaluation was to be cognizant of the requirements and charges mandated for the evaluation (see Appendix A). To augment the overview of the evaluation design presented in Part II, this part of the plan partitions and elaborates the areas of interest laid out in the congressional mandate.

The guiding framework of the program impact pathway is applied to each of these areas, reflecting the committee's understanding of the rationale for how PEPFAR's specific inputs and activities can be plausibly linked to PEPFAR's contribution to effects on HIV-specific health outcomes and impacts. This part of the report illustrates the types of questions that will guide the evaluation of PEPFAR's activities in prevention, adult and pediatric treatment, care and support, child and adolescent wellbeing (including orphans and vulnerable children), and gender-related vulnerability and risk activities. The evaluation will also consider other fundamental activities in the areas of knowledge management and funding flows; these are considered first in this part of the report because they underlie the success of all other programmatic areas. This part of the report culminates with a discussion of cross-cutting activities related to key systems-level goals that are critical for the long term goals articulated by PEPFAR, such as health systems strengthening and transitioning to sustainability and country ownership.

As described in Part II, in each of these areas the evaluation questions will be addressed using a mixed methods approach and layers of investigation and analysis, drawing on a range of available primary and secondary data sources. By applying a mix of methods, data sources, and analytical techniques, the committee will arrive at findings that can be triangulated to draw conclusions about the performance of PEPFAR and its contribution to health impact, even when any one data source is not sufficient or any one methodological approach is not feasible. The extent to which specific methods can be applied to answer the evaluation questions will depend on the timely availability of data that is of sufficient quality to lead to reliable findings. Therefore, the illustrative questions and the methods and data sources that will be used to address them will undergo further refinement and prioritization as a result of the operational planning phase activities described previously.

# SECTION 1: PEPFAR'S KNOWLEDGE MANAGEMENT

The management of knowledge and information is critical to the success of any program because it serves to monitor the activities and effects of the program as well as to guide policies, priorities, and programmatic decisions. Therefore, assessing the performance of PEPFAR's knowledge management activities will be an important part of the evaluation of the performance of PEPFAR as a whole, as well as an assessment of the forward-looking mechanisms that are in place for continuous M&E of the program's progress and appropriate responses.

In PEPFAR I, the primary goal of OGAC's strategic information (SI) efforts for M&E, in partnership with implementing agencies, was to support PEPFAR through results-based planning and implementation, focusing on quality information collection, timely data management and use, evaluation of best practices, and information for decision making. In PEPFAR II, the goals have been expanded to include support of the larger PEPFAR mission. To this end, the expanded SI mission includes building the capacity of countries to improve health outcomes by increasing and strengthening the use of information for effective stewardship of programs and effective implementation of efficient, high-quality, and sustainable health systems (Bouey, 2010).

During PEPFAR II, the SI goals also include improved harmonization of USG reporting needs with country-driven M&E efforts through not only strengthening country capacity and alignment with national data collection, but also through better alignment with global reporting requirements to lessen the burden on implementing partners and partner governments (OGAC, 2009h). An increased focus on both program coverage and quality will be reflected in SI efforts to identify indicators that can give an accurate picture of these two areas (OGAC, 2009d). Finally, although it continues to recognize that PEPFAR is not intended to be a research initiative, the PEPFAR Five-Year Strategy outlines the additional goals of improving the program's efforts to contribute to the evidence base for HIV interventions and to expand the amount of publicly available data (OGAC, 2009g). This expanded research effort will prioritize the evaluation and proactive dissemination of topics that PEPFAR is in a unique position to address as well as studies that focus on methods to improve program delivery (OGAC, 2009h). It will also increase the tracking of outcomes, cost-effectiveness, innovation, and impacts in order to identify timely information regarding the program's effectiveness and impact (OGAC, 2009h).

## Strategic Information Management

Structurally, SI activities at the PEPFAR headquarters level are carried out by USG implementing agencies with coordination through OGAC. These headquarters-level activities draw from a wide range of data-gathering sources (see Figure 5).

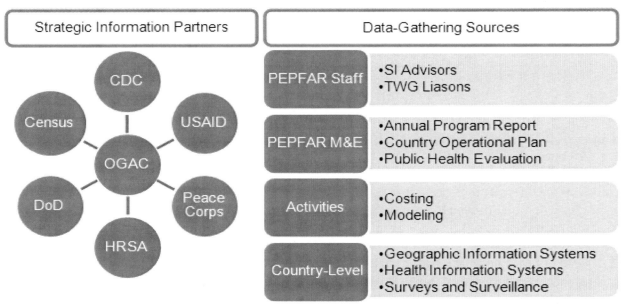

**FIGURE 5** PEPFAR headquarters-level strategic information partners and headquarters-level data-gathering sources.
NOTES: CDC = U.S. Centers for Disease Control and Prevention, Census = U.S. Census Bureau, DoD = U.S. Department of Defense, HRSA = Health Resources and Services Administration of the U.S. Department of Health and Human Services, M&E = monitoring and evaluation, OGAC = Office of the U.S. Global AIDS Coordinator, SI = strategic information, TWG = technical working group, USAID = United States Agency for International Development.
SOURCE: Adapted from Bouey (2010).

The staff at headquarters are responsible for issuing guidance related to COP submission and reporting processes, as well as for providing technical assistance. This guidance instructs country teams on how to successfully complete their reporting requirements. In addition to annual reporting needs, guidance from headquarters can also provide information on collecting, interpreting, and updating basic epidemiologic profiles as well as information on how to develop and incorporate efforts to evaluate new initiatives (OGAC, 2009e). While this guidance focuses primarily on the processes unique to OGAC, it also offers additional information regarding data collection and target setting that has the potential for broader applicability.

Within headquarters there is also a SI technical working group. These efforts at the headquarters level also support M&E activities at the country level through the development of resources such as an M&E Systems Strengthening Tool, which is designed to help partner countries prioritize their M&E needs and encourage alignment with a national M&E strategy, and a Data Quality Assessment Tool (MEASURE Evaluation, 2007; PEPFAR, 2008a).

While management of data collection, storage, and analysis at the country and project level varies, the primary mechanism for reporting and aggregating these data is via an electronic, Internet-based program known as the Country Operational Plan Reporting System (COPRS). Data that are reported via COPRS are collected at the OGAC headquarters level during the relevant semi-annual or annual program reporting periods, depending on the country (OGAC, 2009d). A portion of these data is released to the public and is also communicated to Congress via an annual report. Occasionally, they are used by OGAC to produce additional topic-specific reports (e.g., Report on Gender-Based Violence and HIV/AIDS) (PEPFAR, 2010c). COPRS is currently in transition due to two factors. First, the Next Generation Indicators Reference Guidance was recently released, introducing a limited number of new indicators and redefining some measures that had previously been in use. This guidance was developed in part to support PEPFAR's contribution to global efforts to harmonize reporting requirements for HIV/AIDS initiatives, which aims to reduce the reporting burden of program implementers and to allow more flexibility and increased local ownership of the design of M&E plans (OGAC, 2009d). Second, a new generation of COPRS, COPRS II, is in development and is expected to be deployed in FY2010 (OGAC, 2009e).

## Beyond Information Management

In 2008, PEPFAR began a campaign titled "know your epidemic/know your results" aimed at using information to more closely align program activities with population needs (OGAC, 2008b). As a result, a focus was placed on developing sustainable SI systems to "collect, analyze, critically review, disseminate, interpret, display, and strategically use data at all levels" (OGAC, 2008b). Continuing with this development of SI, the 2009 headquarters operational plan allocated funds for the development of a "draft knowledge management strategy," perhaps in response to the first IOM PEPFAR evaluation recommendation to develop a detailed, overall strategy for institutionalizing its efforts to function as a learning organization and to increase its contributions to the global knowledge base (IOM, 2007; OGAC, 2009f). Coordination among country staff and dissemination of best practices is also facilitated by the PEPFAR implementers' meeting held annually in a PEPFAR country. In addition to sharing information across countries, this meeting includes a variety of breakout sessions dedicated to SI issues (PEPFAR, 2009a).

In addition, as described above, the recent goals for PEPFAR II emphasized the important role of expanding the program's research portfolio to contribute to the publicly available evidence base, with an emphasis on operations research to improve program delivery as well as methods for timely assessments of the program's effectiveness and impact (OGAC, 2009h). Some research activities are already occurring in individual partner countries. For example, the Public Health Evaluations (PHE), initiated in 2007, are a PEPFAR activity intended as a source to inform policy and program-level changes. They currently serve as the primary mechanism through which PEPFAR supports research within countries, including operations research (Edgil, 2010; OGAC, 2009h). Some PHEs are single country, while others are multi-site investigations. The selection of PHE proposals (annually solicited from investigators) is performed by an interagency technical policy group charged with prioritizing areas in need of evaluation, overseeing the implementation of evaluations, and recommending approvals and levels of funding for PHEs. In doing so, priority is given to studies that are driven by locally-identified country needs as well as those that involve local institutions and investigators in the research process.[15] As of 2008 there were 195 PHE activities (Edgil, 2010), with the most recent call for proposals issued by the National Institutes of Health in April 2010.[16]

---

[15] Personal communication from OGAC, April 9, 2010.
[16] *Ibid.*

## PEPFAR's Monitoring and Evaluation Framework

To evaluate PEPFAR's performance in the area of knowledge management, the committee will be guided by the public health questions approach (see Figure 6), a framework that is widely used in the global HIV/AIDS M&E community and has been adopted by OGAC (Bouey, 2010; Rugg et al., 2004; UNAIDS MERG, 2010). The committee will determine the extent to which M&E activities are meeting the goals laid out in this framework and the extent to which these activities are contributing to evaluating and improving the performance of the program and building the capacity of partner countries to use information to improve health outcomes.

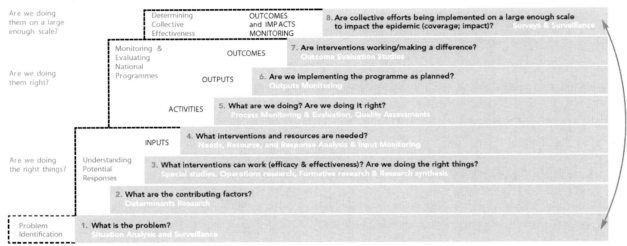

**FIGURE 6** A public health questions approach to HIV monitoring and evaluation.
SOURCE: Reprinted, with permission, from UNAIDS MERG (2010).

## Illustrative Questions

The evaluation of PEPFAR's SI activities will be carried out at the level of headquarters and in those partner countries where PEPFAR has made major investment in M&E. In order to accomplish the assessment, the committee will use a desk review of OGAC and country-level M&E strategy and implementation procedures and data management systems since the beginning of PEPFAR (i.e., including different iterations over time). The committee will also examine M&E funding allocations and expenditures at global and country levels where available. A review of national M&E strategies, national M&E assessment reports, and reports on the HIV epidemic and response, including global reports such as United Nations General Assembly Special Session (UNGASS) documents or M&E data from UNAIDS's National Composite Policy Index, will also provide context for the evaluation.

Due to the limitations in assessing the progress of efforts over time from guidance and assessment documents, the committee will also rely on structured interviews with key SI and programmatic PEPFAR staff at all levels (OGAC, USG agencies, OGAC SI technical working groups, country staff, contractors/implementers) regarding the mechanisms and role of SI in the PEPFAR program and in informing the national HIV response. The committee may also explore structured interviews with key M&E and programmatic staff of each country's national AIDS program as well as other multilateral and bilateral organizations (including UNAIDS, WHO, the

Global Fund) about the role of PEPFAR as a partner at the local, national, and global levels. These interviews could be incorporated as a part of the committee's country visits or conducted by phone or video conference (or alternative self-completed questionnaire) for those countries where a country visit is not planned. The committee's analysis of the completeness and validity of data requested from OGAC and implementing partners for all areas of this evaluation will also inform an assessment of SI and M&E performance and progress.

In order to assess PEPFAR's contribution to the global knowledge base, the committee will assess PEPFAR's participation in international M&E development processes. The committee will also assess current research efforts, such as the PHEs, and associated dissemination efforts, such as presentations from PEPFAR programs at the annual implementers' meeting and other international conferences like the meetings of the International AIDS Society. In addition, a preliminary search of published literature conducted during this planning phase will provide the foundation for a more extensive review during the evaluation of available articles, reports, and other publications resulting from PEPFAR-funded activities.

The following are examples of illustrative questions that the committee may consider in the evaluation. These questions related to knowledge management reflect a fundamental activity of the program and as such are intended to contribute to addressing all of the areas for consideration in the congressional mandate, as described in the Statement of Task (see Appendix A).

*To what extent has investment in M&E resulted in effective systems for PEPFAR decision making and for program management and improvement at both the headquarters and country levels?*

Is data collection and analysis being used for decision making about PEPFAR program priorities, implementation strategies, effectiveness, and efficiency? For example, is PEPFAR using data to support evidence-based COP planning and resource allocation? Does data collection lead to timely identification of implementation problems, and does this result in corrective action? Does data on targets determine whether programs are implemented on a large enough scale to have an impact on the epidemic?

Are the data collated, analyzed, interpreted, presented, and disseminated in a manner that allows for use in decision making? What are the mechanisms used to assure the validity and quality of data? What mechanisms are in place to facilitate the translation of information produced by M&E systems into action? Are lessons learned accessible and are changes applied across the whole of the program where appropriate?

Have operations research and other research activities supported by PEPFAR, such as PHEs, had an impact on service delivery and led to improved outcomes of prevention, treatment, and care programs supported by PEPFAR? Are operations and other research activities using appropriate methodologies and resulting in information that is shared across sites, programs, and countries to optimize and inform policy and program decisions? Are these research activities addressing the issues most in need of evaluation? What should the priorities be for future PHEs and other research activities?

What has been the impact of PEPFAR reporting requirements for accountability purposes (i.e., reporting to the U.S. Congress) on continuation of PEPFAR funding and on decision making for priority investments as well as program management and improvement?

What progress has been made on PEPFAR's intentions to develop indicators where there are currently limited mechanisms for tracking progress, such as gender and health systems strengthening?

Are there sufficient M&E mechanisms and capacity to evaluate whether the program meets new goals for sustainability and country ownership, as well as the resulting outcomes and impact of changes made to address those goals?

Does OGAC draw on sources of data outside of PEPFAR to inform programmatic and policy decisions?

*To what extent is PEPFAR contributing to the global knowledge base?*

Are PEPFAR-funded activities resulting in research that is contributing to the scientific knowledge base? Are research findings, lessons learned, and best practices from PEPFAR available in the published literature? What other mechanisms are used to disseminate knowledge not only within but also beyond PEPFAR? To what extent is that process encouraged or facilitated?

To what extent is PEPFAR engaging with other international stakeholders around SI activities? To what extent is PEPFAR contributing to the development of state-of-the-art practices in M&E at the global level?

*To what extent has PEPFAR built/is PEPFAR building capacity at the country level, including national M&E systems,[17] to support an appropriate, effective, and efficient national HIV response?*

What is PEPFAR's approach to supporting long-term sustainability of the national M&E system? How is PEPFAR translating the commitment of the United States to the "Third One" adopted by most donors—one national M&E system to reduce reporting burden and transactional costs of business for countries with multiple donors?

To what extent is the PEPFAR M&E strategy aligned with and incorporated in the national M&E strategy/plan? What are the positive and negative effects of the headquarters-level PEPFAR M&E strategy on national M&E systems? To what extent and how are PEPFAR M&E data (program planning, routine program

---

[17] National M&E system refers to M&E at the national, sub-national, and service-delivery levels.

monitoring, findings from special studies) shared with the national M&E system to ensure a coordinated HIV response and to guide program improvement?

What mechanisms are used by PEPFAR for M&E capacity building and to ensure effective partnerships for technical cooperation and technology transfer? What are the effects of the PEPFAR M&E capacity building activities on national M&E system strengthening and data use for decision making?

To what extent has PEPFAR built/is PEPFAR building M&E capacity within partner organizations implementing programs at the country level, including data analysis and management?

## SECTION 2: MAPPING PEPFAR FUNDING

All donor-specific impact evaluations are limited by the ability to attribute desired impacts to the investments of a single program given the presence of similar and complementary programs funded by other sources, so the committee's evaluation will focus on PEPFAR's contribution to global efforts to fight HIV/AIDS (IOM, 2008). PEPFAR inputs include policy guidance and regulations, personnel, technical assistance and training, facilities and equipment, knowledge transfer and research, and funding. While all are important to assessing PEPFAR's impact, the level and allocation of funding, as well as how the funding is used, underpins much of the evaluation. It both represents the most direct measure of the USG's investment to address the global AIDS pandemic and provides a critical input needed for answering many of the other evaluation questions pertaining to the impact of PEPFAR. These include questions about PEPFAR's impact on specific health targets, such as reducing HIV incidence, and its impact on broader mandates and goals, such as promoting long-term sustainability, country ownership, and health systems strengthening. As such, financing is a cross-cutting aspect of the overall evaluation, embedded within each of the other main evaluation questions.

To evaluate the impact of PEPFAR's financial investments on desired program impacts, the committee will develop a funding flow framework for PEPFAR financing, designed to map funds throughout the life cycle of the program. It will begin with Congress, which appropriates funding to federal agencies, and follow funding provided by federal agencies to prime partners and other implementers in an attempt to map all the way to service providers in the field and ultimately to beneficiaries. The objective of this financial framework is not to conduct a financial audit but to assess the role of U.S. funding in the context of the overall evaluation of PEPFAR's impact on health and other outcomes and to illustrate the specific points at which the USG intervenes, how it intervenes, and the level of its intervention. Figure 7 represents the committee's initial understanding of the landscape of PEPFAR funding flows, which may change as more information is accumulated throughout the evaluation.

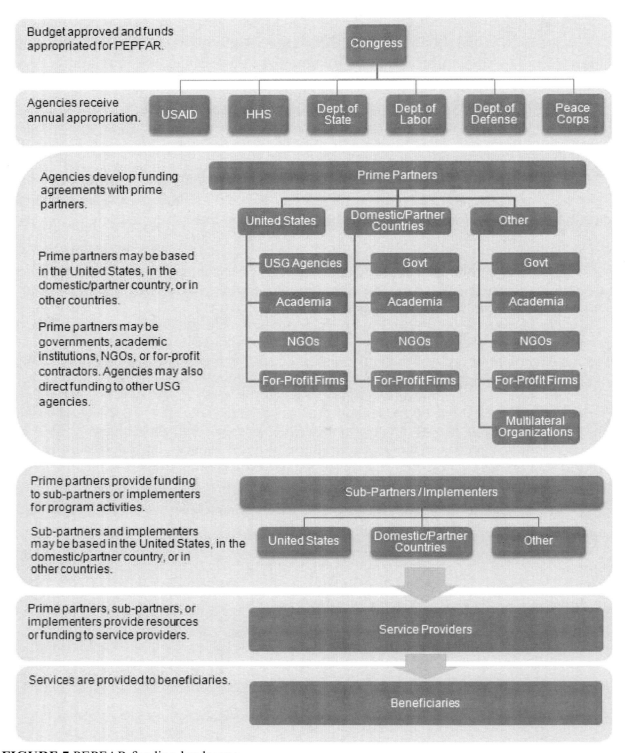

**FIGURE 7** PEPFAR funding landscape.
NOTES: Dept. = department, Govt = government, HHS = U.S. Department of Human Health and Services, NGOs = non-governmental organizations, USAID = U.S. Agency for International Development, USG = U.S. government.
SOURCE: Committee assessment based on a review of documents from OGAC, including PEPFAR operational plans and partner information, as well as other readily available sources.

The evaluation will also situate PEPFAR investments within the larger landscape of investments made by other funders to allow for an assessment of PEPFAR's relative financial contributions to global efforts to combat HIV/AIDS. This is important because nearly all of the countries that receive PEPFAR funding also receive funding for HIV/AIDS programs from other sources (see Table 1 for an illustration of the current funding landscape in PEPFAR countries). The committee will therefore develop another financial framework to situate PEPFAR within the broader funding landscape, designed to capture PEPFAR's relative contribution globally and by country. It will include other donor governments, multilateral institutions, partner country governments and households, and the private sector.

**TABLE 1** Current HIV/AIDS Funding from Select Donors Received by PEPFAR Countries (as of April 2010)

| Country | Multilateral | | Bilateral | |
| --- | --- | --- | --- | --- |
| | Global Fund | World Bank | CIDA | DFID |
| Angola | X | X | X | |
| Botswana | | | | |
| Cambodia | X | X | | X |
| China | X | | | X |
| Congo, Democratic Republic of the | X | X | | X |
| Côte d'Ivoire | X | X | X | |
| Dominican Republic | X | | X | |
| Ethiopia | X | X | X | X |
| Ghana | X | X | X | X |
| Guyana | X | | X | |
| Haiti | X | | X | |
| India | X | X | X | X |
| Indonesia | X | | | X |
| Kenya | X | X | X | X |
| Lesotho | X | X | | X |
| Malawi | X | X | X | X |
| Mozambique | X | X | X | X |
| Namibia | X | X | | |
| Nigeria | X | X | | X |
| Russia | X | | X | |
| Rwanda | X | X | X | X |
| South Africa | X | | X | X |
| Sudan | X | X | X | |
| Swaziland | X | | X | X |
| Tanzania | X | X | X | X |
| Thailand | X | | | |
| Uganda | X | X | X | X |
| Ukraine | X | | X | |
| Vietnam | X | X | | X |
| Zambia | X | X | | X |
| Zimbabwe | X | | X | X |

NOTE: An X denotes that a country receives or has recently received approval for an HIV/AIDS grant from the Global Fund, or has at least one currently operational HIV/AIDS program funded by the World Bank (excluding IBRD-financed loans), the Canadian International Development Agency (CIDA), or the UK Department for International Development (DFID). CIDA and DFID are representative of other bilateral funders of global HIV/AIDS programming, and the UK in particular is the second largest bilateral donor to HIV/AIDS (Kates et al., 2009).
SOURCE: Compiled from GFATM (2010a), World Bank (2010), CIDA (2010), and DFID (2010).

Finally, since the data used to populate the financial framework are critical inputs for each program area, the committee will attempt, where feasible, to use these data to answer questions surrounding program efficiency, economies of scale, costs of intermediate units of analysis (e.g., the unit cost of outputs, the costs per beneficiary), and costs per intermediate outcomes (e.g., school enrollment, change in condom use, persons on treatment, and child infections averted from PMTCT, etc.). Ultimately, the framework proposed here will be designed to provide policymakers with a direct measure of PEPFAR's impact on the global HIV/AIDS epidemic.

## Illustrative Questions

The committee will consult a variety of data sources including PEPFAR and USG agencies (e.g., OGAC databases, COPs, partnership frameworks, prime and sub-prime partner reports, etc.), other donors and international stakeholders (UNAIDS, the World Bank, the Global Fund, Organisation for Economic Co-operation and Development [OECD], etc.), partner countries, and the relevant evaluation literature. To identify data sources and availability, the committee will need to conduct structured interviews with relevant stakeholders including USG representatives, implementers, partners, and others. Data collection and quality will be a primary potential limitation since much of the analysis is predicated on being able to obtain timely data from these sources. The complexities of mapping financing flows from multiple donors to multiple countries will also complicate the ability to access consistent and complete longitudinal data.

Given the timely availability of quality data, the following are examples of illustrative questions that are feasible to address. These questions related to the flow of funding reflect a fundamental aspect of program operations and as such are intended to contribute to addressing all of the areas for consideration in the congressional mandate, as described in the Statement of Task (see Appendix A).

*How much PEPFAR funding is provided and what is its relative contribution to global efforts against HIV/AIDS?*

Where possible, the committee will use longitudinal data to analyze PEPFAR's relative contribution over time and determine whether PEPFAR has been able to leverage additional resources from other donors and national governments. To further describe the contribution of PEPFAR funding, the committee will attempt to determine the proportion of the national budget and the gross domestic product that would need to be spent on health and HIV/AIDS if partner governments were to take on these expenditures.

*How is PEPFAR funding provided to partner countries and USG partners?*

Initially, the committee will analyze COPs and partnership frameworks to identify a general mapping of funding flows and seek to characterize countries according to a sub-set of different types of models or frameworks. The committee aims to determine whether PEPFAR funding is provided through bilateral or multilateral channels and which mechanisms are used to deliver funding, such as cash transfers or commodities. To further describe funding cascades, the committee will attempt an analysis of PEPFAR's disbursement procedures to determine how quickly funding is provided to the field once it has been appropriated by Congress, obligated to countries, and disbursed to partners.

*Who are the recipients of PEPFAR funding at each stage of program?*

As depicted in Figure 8, PEPFAR channels funding through governments, NGOs, academic institutions, and private contractors that may be based in the United States, in partner countries, or in other countries. The committee will seek to analyze the proportion of funding that flows to each type of recipient and analyze longitudinal trends. A preliminary committee analysis of FY2008 obligations to prime partners identified three main sub-types when stratified by geographic location and five sub-types when stratified by geographic location and organizational type, as follows (listed in order of share of investment):

Prime Partner Funding Flow Sub-Types by Geographic Location
1.  United States
2.  Domestic/Partner Country
3.  Other/International

Prime Partner Funding Flow Sub-Types by Geographic Location and Organizational Type
1.  U.S. NGO
2.  U.S. Academic
3.  Domestic/Partner Country NGO
4.  Domestic/Partner Country Government
5.  U.S. for Profit Firms

The relative distribution of funds by agency origin (United States versus partner country) and by sector (government, NGO, academia, private sector) *over time* also will be assessed. Understanding these patterns may help elucidate the degree to which the targeting of funding supports, or potentially undercuts, the goal of increasing country ownership of HIV programming. The criteria for providing grants to local implementing partners and how they are monitored may also contribute to an assessment of whether this process contributes to the goals of increasing country ownership. In addition, the performance of the prime partner organizations in terms of accountability, administrative transparency, and good governance could be additional metrics to consider in the evaluation.

Finally, assessing the distribution of funding in this way may help to provide data and information on the amount of funding that actually reaches the field after accounting for intermediaries along the way.

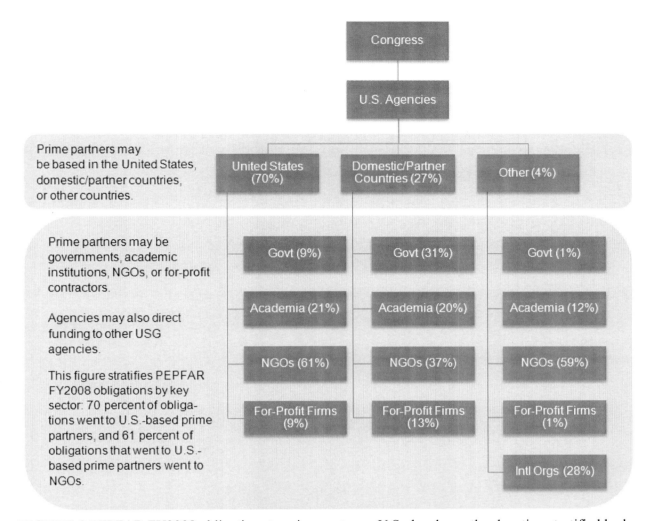

**FIGURE 8** PEPFAR FY2008 obligations to prime partners: U.S., local, or other location stratified by key sector.

NOTES: Totals do not equal 100 percent due to rounding. Govt = government, Intl = international, NGOs = non-governmental organization, Orgs = organizations.

SOURCE: Preliminary committee analysis based on FY2008 OGAC data on obligations to prime partners available at http://www.pepfar.gov/partners/index.htm.

*How are PEPFAR funds distributed among different programmatic areas and interventions?*

*How are funds from PEPFAR and the Global Fund meshed together in countries? Are the joint funds maximized for service delivery and coverage?*

The committee will seek to measure the proportion of funding spent in each program area, such as prevention, treatment, care and support, and health systems. Within each program area, the committee will attempt to identify the level of funding for specific interventions and analyze PEPFAR's efforts to allocate funding appropriately based on country needs and available evidence. In order to analyze whether efficiencies are being achieved, the committee will attempt to determine the unit costs of key PEPFAR interventions and how they vary by type of intervention, country, and other variables of interest.

*Which populations are supported through PEPFAR funding?*

In order to evaluate the impact of PEPFAR funding, the committee will seek to determine the specific populations, such as women, children, and other vulnerable populations, reached with program interventions. The committee will use existing data from reliable sources to measure the number of people living with HIV/AIDS (PLWHA) and compare to the number of vulnerable people reached through PEPFAR programming. The number and types of populations supported by PEPFAR funding will be measured through quantitative analysis of PEPFAR indicators. Aggregated data reported to OGAC provide limited insight about the types of populations supported, so the committee will seek disaggregated data from other sources.

## SECTION 3: PREVENTION SERVICES

It has been estimated that a new HIV infection occurs globally every 12 seconds, and there is agreement that in most countries incident infections are outpacing the number of people placed on ART (Global HIV Prevention Working Group, 2010; UNAIDS and WHO, 2009; Zachariah et al., 2010). At the same time, HIV prevention budgets have been falling in several countries. Currently there is an increasing push by the global community to scale up effective, evidence-based prevention strategies with the knowledge that averting new infections is the only way to bend the curve of the epidemic. Information about new behavioral, biomedical, and structural prevention approaches is growing and individual countries, regions, or localities are being encouraged to incorporate all of the approaches into a comprehensive strategy. PEPFAR is collaborating with WHO and UNAIDS in these efforts and the program's prevention goals, if attained, are intended to help address these deficits.

This section describes the current state of the program's prevention efforts and some of the potential questions and challenges under consideration by the committee to evaluate the extent to which PEPFAR I and II have met their prevention targets and goals. In addition to PEPFAR I's original prevention performance target, there was also the country target of reducing expected HIV incidence by 50 percent (IOM, 2007).

In PEPFAR I, the prevention target was to be achieved through five funding and reporting subcategories: Abstinence/be faithful, Condoms and other prevention (e.g., IDU, military forces, street children), PMTCT, Blood safety, and Injection safety (IOM, 2007). The prevention activities undertaken that correspond to those funding and reporting categories were: promotion of behavior change aimed at risk avoidance and reduction, comprehensive programs for people who engage in high-risk behavior, PMTCT services, and reduction of medical transmission of HIV by ensuring safe blood supplies (OGAC, 2004).

PEPFAR II promotes a transition to increasingly country-owned HIV programs that adequately address their HIV epidemics over time, including expanding prevention in both concentrated and generalized epidemics. The are several targets for PEPFAR II: to support the prevention of more than 12 million infections over the course of the entire program (since 2003),[18] to ensure that every partner country with a generalized epidemic has both 80 percent coverage of testing for pregnant women at the national level[19] and 85 percent coverage of ARV drug prophylaxis and treatment of women found to be HIV-infected (OGAC, 2009g), to double the number of at-risk babies born HIV-free from the 240,000 babies of HIV-positive mothers who were born HIV-negative during the first five years of PEPFAR (OGAC, 2009g), and lastly to provide 100 percent of youth in PEPFAR prevention programs, in every partner country with a generalized epidemic, with comprehensive and correct knowledge of the ways HIV is transmitted and ways to protect themselves, consistent with Millennium Development Goals (MDGs) indicators in this area (OGAC, 2009g).

The Lantos–Hyde Act of 2008 requires the Coordinator to establish a balanced HIV sexual transmission prevention strategy to govern expenditures for prevention activities in countries with generalized epidemics. This "balanced funding" directive replaces the "one-third abstinence or be faithful" budget earmark requirement in the original 2003 legislation. Instead of identifying a specific requirement for the distribution of sexual prevention funds, countries are

---

[18] *Supra.*, note 6 at §301(a)(2), 22 U.S.C. §2151b-2(b)(1)(A)(i).
[19] *Ibid.*, §301(a)(2), 22 U.S.C. §2151b-2(b)(1)(A)(iv).

now required to provide a compelling explanation, justified by the Coordinator, if less than 50 percent of this funding is directed toward activities promoting (a) abstinence, (b) delay of sexual debut, (c) monogamy, (d) fidelity, and (e) partner reduction. The Coordinator is also required to annually publish, and make available to the public, a report that details the progress toward implementation of this prevention strategy (OGAC, 2009e). Similarly, research and dissemination of best practices in prevention methodology have also been identified as priorities for PEPFAR II (OGAC, 2009i).

In addition to the performance targets, PEPFAR II has also established additional overarching goals for prevention, such as strengthening partner country capacity to generate and use timely, accurate, and up-to-date epidemiological information (emphasizing prevention efforts targeted toward most vulnerable populations); encouraging use of innovative strategies for data mapping and service provision; and developing goals for each individual prevention category (OGAC, 2009h).

## Objective and Scope

Evaluation of PEPFAR's efforts toward prevention and assessment of any impacts they may have had are essential to understanding if PEPFAR is meeting its targets of averting more than 12 million new infections. The committee will evaluate the extent to which PEPFAR is effectively engaging in scale-up of combinations of evidence-based HIV prevention intervention. The categories of PEPFAR prevention interventions are shown in Table 2.

**TABLE 2** Categories of PEPFAR Prevention Interventions

|  | **Behavioral** | **Structural** | **Biomedical** |
|---|---|---|---|
| Prevention of Mother To Child Transmission | Improving awareness and acceptability of HIV testing and antiretroviral drug use in pregnancy | Increasing access to HIV testing and antiretroviral drugs during pregnancy | Administration of antiretroviral drugs during pregnancy, at birth and breastfeeding |
| Blood Safety | Education about (in) appropriate use of transfusion | Developing a national transfusion policy Ensuring continual access to blood screening supplies | Screening blood prior to transfusion |
| Injecting Drug Use | Youth education to reduce injecting drug use initiation | Increasing access to drug treatment services or clean needles | Methadone and buprenorphine |
| Sexual | Counseling to reduce concurrency, inconsistent condom use, HIV education for youth | Sex education in schools to delay sexual debut | Male circumcision |
| Prevention in People Living with HIV/AIDS | Counseling to increase condom use and reduce concurrency | Incorporating trained counselors in treatment centers | Testing partners to detect discordancy and identification and treatment of sexually transmitted infections and opportunistic infections |

NOTE: Needle or syringe exchange programs (NSPs) have been shown to be an evidence-based method to reduce HIV and other blood-borne pathogens (IOM, 2006). The ban on domestic funding for NSPs was lifted by the U.S. Congress as part of the FY2010 appropriations process. No similar ban was codified for international assistance accounts (Consolidated Appropriations Act, 2010, P.L. 3288-2, 111th Congress, 1st Session, [January 6, 2009]). However, "foreign affairs programs, including PEPFAR, have traditionally followed the domestic policy guidance regarding NSPs" (Personal communication from OGAC, January 8, 2010). OGAC reports that this lifted ban creates an opportunity for PEPFAR's MARP TWG to explore ways to support NSPs as part of a comprehensive package of services for IDUs and to develop a revised set of comprehensive guidance for PEPFAR programs and teams so that NSPs can augment prevention, treatment, and care activities already provided to this population (Personal communication from OGAC, January 8, 2010).

*Gateway Activities Targeting Prevention That Will Be Examined and Used For Analysis*

In addition to specific interventions, there are additional gateway activities related to PEPFAR's prevention efforts. These gateway activities do not, in and of themselves, reduce the number of new infections, but are critical to targeting prevention services and monitoring the effects and impact of interventions on the prevention goal of reducing new infections. They include HIV testing and counseling in both the community and clinic settings and surveillance activities in general and sub-populations.

*Challenges in Prevention Implementation*

Implementation of programs for HIV prevention face many challenges related to context, culture, and information. The gateway activity of surveillance and the use of spatial mapping tools (e.g. Geographical Information Systems) to describe or visually represent epidemics are critically important, as many countries do not have a clear picture of their epidemic at the national, regional, or local levels. While a sufficient understanding of the nature of the epidemic can more effectively guide programmatic decisions to target appropriate population groups, in some countries multiple types of epidemics are occurring simultaneously both within and across different regions. This poses challenges during the development of an HIV prevention strategic plan and requires more complicated combinations of activities that increase the number of logistic and coordination barriers to be managed. Finally, varying types of stigma and discrimination can restrict the ability of prevention programs to reach at-risk and vulnerable populations such as IDUs, CSWs, and women and girls. Each of these issues provide context when evaluating the areas of success and failure in PEPFAR's prevention efforts (OGAC, 2009i).

## Program Impact Pathway

PEPFAR's prevention efforts will be assessed in accordance with a program impact pathway framework, as shown in Figure 9. The evaluation will draw on a variety of data sources, including outputs and outcomes as measured by PEPFAR countries and OGAC. For estimating the impact measure of incidence, the committee will consider emerging globally accepted proxy measures, such as prevalence in young people, as well U.S. Census Bureau and other modeling efforts. The committee may also use available data to consult with experts who model infections averted for PEPFAR in particular. Since prevalence is affected by incidence, duration (longevity should increase with more people getting on ART), and population growth, the committee will be interested to know how the modelers will parse out these relative constituents. While there is concern about relying too heavily on these statistical forecasts, the committee feels that models have utility. They will be examined taking into account their limitations, which are primarily determined by the quality of the data available to do the modeling. The evaluation may also assess the contribution that PEPFAR funds made to achieve impact at the country level by undertaking a trend analysis of incidence figures over time and comparing that to key policy or program or funding events that occurred over the same time period.

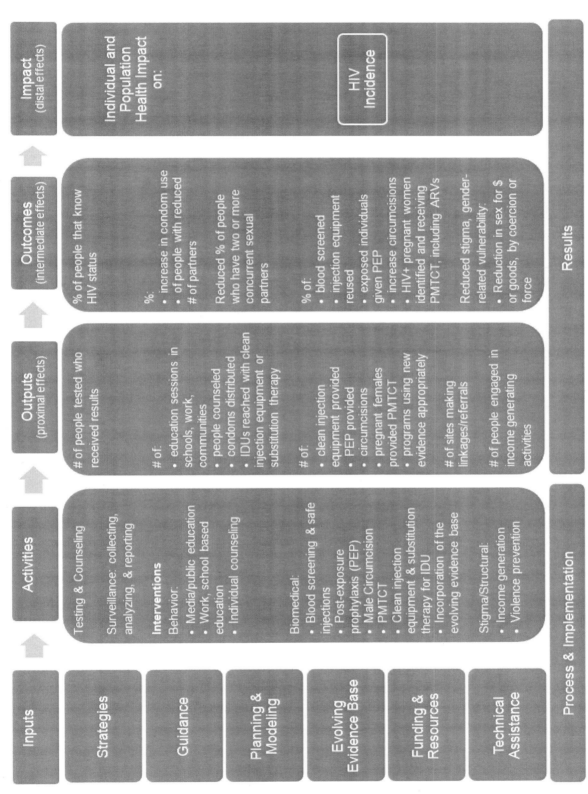

**FIGURE 9** Program impact pathway for evaluation of PEPFAR's prevention programs.
NOTES: ARVs = antiretroviral drugs, IDU = injecting drug user, PMTCT = prevention of mother-to-child transmission.

**Illustrative Questions**

To assess whether both PEPFAR I and II have achieved their prevention goals, the committee will not only evaluate whether they met their quantitative targets, but also assess whether in doing so, they provided quality services, met the needs of the countries in which programs were implemented, and met their own overarching goals (coordination, integration, health system strengthening, and building capacity) as articulated in the strategy for PEPFAR II (OGAC, 2009g).

The evaluation of PEPFAR's prevention efforts, outputs, and outcomes is subject to a variety of limitations including the quality and timely availability of quality data. In addition, as a part of OGAC's Next Generation Indicators project, many of the indicators centrally collected by OGAC that are applicable to prevention efforts were modified or revised at the end of 2009, which may affect the ability of the committee to assess temporal trends or compare original PEPFAR countries with those added more recently. Each individual topic also contains its own challenges and limitations that may limit the committee's analysis; these are discussed below. The following illustrative questions are intended to contribute to addressing part A, item ii and part B, items i and v of the areas for consideration in the congressional mandate.[20]

*Are prevention strategies for a country defined based on an epidemiological analysis and evidence of what works?*

*Has PEPFAR supported routine behavioral and epidemiological surveillance at the country level to identify sub-national variations in at-risk groups and used these data to target prevention interventions to appropriate groups (most-at-risk populations, other vulnerable populations, youth and adolescents, adults)?*

*Is PEPFAR appropriately and efficiently incorporating emerging evidence on prevention techniques into its programmatic guidance?*

Surveillance strategies can include both biomedical and behavioral measures to determine disease prevalence (using HIV testing data including antenatal and at-risk populations), seroincidence (using "detuned" assays such as BED[21] in population surveys), and risk behavior prevalence (via Demographic and Health Surveys [DHS] or "second generation" surveys). The frequency with which these types of data-gathering methods occur, the methods through which PEPFAR supports their implementation, and the dissemination and use of the data obtained will be assessed by the committee. This will be done by relying on publicly available data sets from DHS and other population surveys as well as qualitative data gathered through site visit interviews. PEPFAR indicators and programmatic guidance related to prevention efforts will be coupled with data from other sources on the nature of the national epidemics and on internationally-accepted best practices for HIV prevention. Studies on the efficacy of new

---

[20] (A)(ii) an evaluation of the impact on health of prevention, treatment, and care efforts that are supported by United States funding, including multilateral and bilateral programs involving joint operations
(B)(i) an assessment of progress toward prevention, treatment, and care targets
(B)(v) an evaluation of the impact of prevention programs on HIV incidence in relevant population groups
[21] *Supra.*, note 12.

approaches to HIV prevention such as pre-exposure prophylaxis (PrEP), microbicides, and vaccine are under way, therefore these types of interventions would not be part of this evaluation (OGAC, 2009i).

> *How does the distribution of funding for prevention activities compare to the epidemiology of the local epidemic? What is PEPFAR's progress toward the development and implementation of a prevention strategy and balanced funding portfolio? How is prevention funding, for countries and OGAC, aligned with elements of the prevention strategy?*

As a backdrop to the evaluation of outcomes and impact, the evaluation may also determine the percentage of funds spent by PEPFAR I and II (by year) on prevention overall, by subcategories, by region, and within countries. The subcategory expenditures can be examined by the committee to determine whether they match with the estimated populations at risk in the country to provide an assessment of the country's ability or willingness to adhere to the guidance of OGAC in "know your epidemic/know your results" and to fund correspondingly appropriate activities. This new guidance from OGAC has resulted in headquarter-suggested realignment of funds in the country when there are significant mismatches (Moloney-Kitts, 2009). In addition, the committee will attempt to determine the funding for each region and country by the prevalence by year and by sub-population. Expenditure studies should also compare the level of investment in prevention activities and the types of programs supported by country and by implementing partners, as well as whether these factors are associated with achievement of prevention objectives. Given the sensitivity surrounding programmatic financial data, the committee anticipates there will be difficulty regarding availability for a complete assessment. The committee will seek whatever data and information are available from OGAC to assess the progress on the development and implementation of the described prevention strategy and its programmatic and budgetary elements, as well as the interaction between this legislative guidance and PEPFAR's stated goal of mapping each country's epidemic and aligning prevention responses to the identified needs (OGAC, 2009g).

> *Within each country, have HIV prevention programs reached the performance targets for prevention for both PEPFAR I and II? Is coverage of each service or a combination of services expanding over time?*

Progress toward the targets previously outlined will be assessed primarily using aggregated indicators that are reported to OGAC. These are available for the majority of the targets. However, for some areas, such as behavior change communication (BCC), additional PEPFAR indicators not reported to OGAC will also be required in order to address the question more completely. The committee will also attempt to assess PEPFAR's progress toward its stated goals in each of the specific prevention areas. For many of these goals for which no reported indicators exists at the aggregated headquarters level at OGAC, the committee will focus on qualitative primary data collection during site visits and will seek out additional quantitative data where available.

> *Has the number of people who have been counseled and tested and received their results increased over time?*

*Have counseling and testing services been offered in an equitable way to women (pregnant and non-pregnant) and men, to young people as well as adults, and to locally-identified vulnerable populations?*

To address PEPFAR's efforts toward expanding its counseling and testing services, the committee will analyze the reported PEPFAR indicators regarding the number of people who receive counseling and testing services and their results. While this indicator is disaggregated by sex, it may be insufficient to identify if programs are reaching all of the at-risk populations in need or if counseling and testing programs are successfully linking with intervention facilities. Where this is the case, the committee will pursue other sources of quantitative and qualitative data.

*What are the effects of the behavioral interventions (education and awareness, condom education and distribution, peer education, sex and HIV prevention education, group and individual behavioral interventions, etc.) that are being implemented?*

BCC programs occur in multiple settings and may be targeted to general population participants or specific at-risk groups. The committee will use indicators aggregated and reported to OGAC regarding number and types of individuals reached with BCC programs, as well as the disaggregation of these indicators where available. These indicators cover the range and frequency of behavior change programs, but do not sufficiently address the effectiveness of these programs with respect to whether the participants actually changed their behavior following the activity. To try to look longitudinally at prevalence as a reflection of the outcome of behavior change efforts, the committee will examine the utility of data from the antenatal population. Potential data sources include large international NGOs that have programs in many PEPFAR countries and therefore have very large cohorts across multiple countries. Some data may also be obtained through consultation with modelers. However, in general the committee will have limited ability to address this effectiveness issue.

*What has been the coverage and outcome or impact of biomedical prevention interventions, which include blood safety, PMTCT, PEP, and male circumcision? How has PMTCT been maximized with jointly operated activities between PEPFAR and the Global Fund? How has coverage expanded as result of joint efforts?*

Implementation and tracking of biomedical prevention programs varies significantly and targets a broad range of individuals at all ages. Data for the evaluation of biomedical prevention interventions will be obtained from aggregated OGAC level indicators and other sources at the country and local levels, as there are not reported PEPFAR indicators for blood safety, PEP, and male circumcision. Challenges associated with evaluating these interventions also include emerging knowledge and best practices that will have to be incorporated in the future and may alter the trajectory of affected programs. This information may be supplemented by qualitative data collected during site visits.

*Are successful linkages being developed between PEPFAR prevention services and other services where appropriate in order to better meet the needs of targeted individuals and to increase coverage and efficiencies when available? For example, are women identified as HIV-positive and HIV-exposed infants in PMTCT programs successfully referred to and enrolled in treatment programs?*

Prevention services have the potential to serve as entry points to identify those in need and increase access for treatment and other services. Optimal implementation of PMTCT programs, for example, can not only reduce perinatal transmission to 2 percent with the use of combination ART, regimens but also serve as a linkage to provide HIV-positive women with ART (Cunningham et al., 2002; Dorenbaum et al., 2002; Kuhn et al., 2008).

As there are currently no centrally reported indicators for "linkages or referrals," the committee will rely primarily on recommended measures such as "the number of health facilities providing antenatal care that provide both HIV and PMTCT services on site" as well as information collected during country site visits. The committee may also attempt to triangulate, where available, the information collected with indicators on PMTCT services coverage and ART coverage for women in specific regions, in order to gain insight into PEPFAR's progress toward its goal of 85 percent prophylaxis and treatment of pregnant women found to be HIV-positive.

*Has PEPFAR implemented effective prevention programs for injecting and other drug users (behavioral, biomedical, and structural interventions and approaches) in regions/countries where drug use drives the epidemic? What has been their effect? What has been the coverage and are interventions evidence-based?*

The committee will use the reported PEPFAR output indicator of "number of [IDUs] on opioid substitution therapy" and the recommended indicator of "percent of [IDUs] on opioid substitution therapy" where available. However, as more information will likely be required to perform a sufficient evaluation, the committee will also pursue alternative data sources. Issues of stigma and confidentiality pose challenges to program implementation and data collection as the population of IDUs is often hidden or difficult to access.

*In order to increase access to services and adoption of testing and preventive behaviors, what efforts has PEPFAR made to reduce stigma through community programs or campaigns or policy initiatives? What has been their effect?*

Structural and policy approaches to reduce stigma and vulnerability are important components of comprehensive HIV combination prevention, but their outcomes, effects, and impact are difficult to evaluate. The committee will use PEPFAR indicators that are disaggregated by sex and testing location (to avoid obscuring the potential male dominance in results outside of maternal and child health settings) where available and supplement these with qualitative data collected during site visits. However, given the lack of data availability, the potential for analysis of interventions to reduce stigma and vulnerability may be limited.

# SECTION 4: ADULT AND PEDIATRIC TREATMENT

Recognizing the need for delivering life-saving treatment to the millions of people living with HIV as a global health emergency, PEPFAR I strategically focused on the rapid scale-up of HIV treatment services and an increase in the coverage of HIV-infected individuals in need of ART (IOM, 2007). As of September 30, 2009, PEPFAR has contributed to the support of treatment for 2,485,300 people, of which 8 percent are children under 15 years of age, through bilateral programs in countries (OGAC, 2010). As shown in Table 3, in 2008 PEPFAR reached the legislative 5-year target of assuring treatment for 2 million people (PEPFAR, 2009c), which included treatment for 131,500 children under 15 years of age (OGAC, 2009c). Since this contribution "has been the major success of PEPFAR" scale-up efforts in the early years (OGAC, 2009i, p. 26), PEPFAR II (2009–2013) plans will focus on supporting a country-led response to the HIV/AIDS epidemic, especially assisting countries in identifying resources available, increasing country coverage, and prioritizing the unmet needs for ART for PLWHA.

**TABLE 3** Cumulative Number of People on Antiretroviral Treatment by PEPFAR Country

| Country | PEPFAR Five-Year Target (2003-2008)[a] | FY2005 | FY2006 | FY2007 | FY2008 |
|---|---|---|---|---|---|
| Botswana[b] | 33,000 | 37,300 | 67,500 | 90,500 | 111,700 |
| Côte d'Ivoire | 77,000 | 11,100 | 27,600 | 46,000 | 50,500 |
| Ethiopia | 210,000 | 16,200 | 40,000 | 81,800 | 119,600 |
| Guyana | 2,000 | 800 | 1,600 | 2,100 | 2,300 |
| Haiti | 25,000 | 4,300 | 8,000 | 12,900 | 17,700 |
| Kenya | 250,000 | 44,700 | 97,800 | 166,400 | 229,700 |
| Mozambique | 110,000 | 16,200 | 34,200 | 78,200 | 118,000 |
| Namibia | 23,000 | 14,300 | 26,300 | 43,700 | 56,100 |
| Nigeria | 350,000 | 28,500 | 67,100[c] | 126,400 | 211,500 |
| Rwanda | 50,000 | 15,900 | 30,000 | 44,400 | 59,900 |
| South Africa | 500,000 | 93,000 | 210,300 | 329,000 | 549,700 |
| Tanzania | 150,000 | 14,700 | 44,300 | 96,700 | 144,100 |
| Uganda | 60,000 | 67,500 | 89,200 | 106,000 | 145,000 |
| Vietnam | 22,000 | 700 | 6,600 | 11,700 | 24,500 |
| Zambia | 120,000 | 36,000 | 71,500 | 122,700 | 167,500 |
| **Total** | **2,000,000** | **401,200** | **822,000** | **1,358,500** | **2,007,800** |

NOTES: Numbers reflect totals of downstream (direct) and upstream (indirect) results.

[a]Based on PEPFAR's Congressional Report to Congress of persons on antiretroviral therapy in the original 15 focus countries as of September 30, 2008.

[b]Botswana results are attributed to the National HIV Program. Beginning FY2006, U.S. Government (USG) downstream contributions in Botswana are embedded in the upstream numbers, following a consensus reached between the USG and the Government of Botswana to report single upstream figures for each relevant indicator.

[c]In Nigeria, it is currently unknown if the government's number of people on treatment accounts for people who are lost to follow up, therefore the total number of people on treatment had been reduced by 15 percent to account for the estimated attrition.

SOURCE: PEPFAR (2009c).

For treatment programs, the host government may use Global Fund, other donor, or country resources to support specific components of services in some PEPFAR treatment sites, while PEPFAR supports other essential components of the treatment services. Beyond these joint operations of treatment sites by PEPFAR and other donors, other support to PEPFAR specific sites may be national or regional in nature (PEPFAR and USAID, 2007). At the same time, in countries where multiple funders (e.g., PEPFAR and the Global Fund) are present, some PEPFAR delivery sites also receive support from other bilateral and multilateral funding through their investments in the government's national HIV/AIDS programs. From 2005–2009, the total number of individuals directly supported on ART that counted toward the 5-year legislative target included the estimated overlap of individuals receiving ART with support by both PEPFAR and the Global Fund. As of September 30, 2009, the overlap estimate was 1.3 million individuals (OGAC, 2010). This overlap estimate also is included in the treatment results reported by the Global Fund (2.5 million individuals receiving ART with support from the Global Fund).

To estimate this overlap, PEPFAR conducts a review of the treatment and funding data with the Global Fund and WHO, on a country-by-country basis. In its review, PEPFAR and the Global Fund take into account the percentage or level of contribution to the national HIV/AIDS program in order to determine where there is likely to be overlap (GFTAM, 2009; OGAC, 2010; PEPFAR, 2010b). In FY2009, PEPFAR and the Global Fund directly supported approximately 3.6 million individuals on ART (number of unique individuals supported by PEPFAR and the Global Fund, excluding the estimated overlap). PEPFAR plans to continue to work with the Global Fund to refine attribution methodologies in relation to treatment results (PEPFAR, 2010).

Globally, the efforts in expanding the availability of ARV drugs has resulted in a greater proportion of people living with HIV in need of treatment receiving ART, which is helping to lower HIV-related mortality in multiple countries and regions (UNAIDS and WHO, 2009). Particularly, there is increasing evidence of the effectiveness of ART in decreasing morbidity and mortality in PLWHA in resource-poor settings (Bussmann et al., 2008; Herbst et al., 2009; Jahn et al., 2008; Mermin et al., 2008). Access to ARV drugs in low- and middle-income countries increased 10-fold between 2003 and 2008 (UNAIDS and WHO, 2009). In 2008, ART coverage in low- and middle-income countries reached 42 percent of the 9.5 million people in need, while coverage for children was 38 percent among 730,000 children (WHO et al., 2009). Despite progress in scaling-up access to ART in these countries, the majority of PLWHA and in need of treatment are currently not receiving such services, specifically in sub-Saharan Africa, where there is the greatest need (WHO et al., 2009).

As noted above, in 2008 nearly two-thirds of the children under 15 years of age living with HIV worldwide in need of ART are still not receiving treatment (WHO et al., 2009). Some of the challenges in achieving greater coverage of treatment services for children include availability of cluster of differentiation (CD4) testing and ART at primary care, antenatal, delivery, and postnatal facilities where most maternal-child health care takes place (WHO et al., 2009). Furthermore, the difficulty of early infant diagnosis of HIV (EID), mainly due to the lack of affordable and accessible diagnostic testing and monitoring and to the shortage of ART regimens for children, poses particular challenges for increasing ART coverage among HIV-exposed or HIV-infected infants (UNAIDS, 2008; WHO et al., 2009). Without treatment, HIV infection in children follows an aggressive course including a faster progression to AIDS and death than in adults (Newell et al., 2004; Violari et al., 2008). With approximately 6 percent of PLWHA being children (UNAIDS and WHO, 2009), the disease is disproportionately killing more children than adults even though current WHO guidelines indicate that all HIV-infected infants and children less than 2 years of age should be started on ART immediately upon diagnosis, irrespective of CD4 count or WHO clinical stage (WHO, 2010). In 2008, 14 percent of AIDS-related deaths (280,000) were in children under 15 years of age (UNAIDS and WHO, 2009).

Improved access to pediatric treatment (which includes children 0–14 years) will depend on the ability to identify women and children routinely through maternal-child care service entry points. For example, scaling up optimal implementation of PMTCT programs not only can improve treatment for women by providing HIV-positive pregnant women with ART, but also has the potential to identify and increase access for children in need of HIV treatment services.

WHO revised its ART recommendations in 2009 and is now recommending that ART be initiated at a higher CD4 threshold of 350 cells/mm$^3$ (compared to previous levels of 250 cells/mm$^3$) for all HIV-positive patients, including pregnant women, regardless of the symptoms (WHO, 2009a, 2009b, 2009c). The 2009 WHO ART treatment guidelines for adults and adolescents, however, adds another 50 percent to those in need of ART from the 2008 figure above—increasing this number to approximately 15 million people, which is almost half of the PLWHA worldwide (De Lay, 2010).

In the past 6 years, PEPFAR has supported activities for building laboratory capacity (OGAC, 2006a, 2009a, 2009c), including laboratory equipment, training, and quality control, given that laboratory monitoring is used by clinicians to track key patient outcomes, including the effects of ART on the well-being of a patient (WHO, 2006b, 2007b). Both CD4 and viral load testing, when available, are now recommended under the new 2009 WHO ART guidelines as part of program M&E activities to ensure quality HIV treatment programs (WHO, 2009a, 2009b, 2009c). In many developed countries this is part of the standard patient treatment monitoring; however, there are challenges to implementing CD4 cell and viral load testing in resource-limited settings, including both test cost and lack of infrastructure. These challenges may result in countries making determinations about how high a priority current ART programs should put on making these tests available vis-à-vis expanding the number of patients on treatment (Phillips and van Oosterhout, 2010). There is some evidence that the use of viral load monitoring in resource-limited settings improves patient outcomes as much as it does in high-resource settings (Gupta et al., 2009). The effect of routine CD4 cell monitoring on mortality was modest in a randomized trial in Uganda and Zimbabwe, and thus it requires additional evaluation (Dart Trial Team, 2009).

The expanding goals of ART are to drive and maintain HIV-1 RNA plasma levels below limits of detection, preserve and restore immune function, and prevent or delay the clinical progression of disease (Hammer, 2010). Minimizing drug toxicities and prevention of drug resistance are also important goals of ART, and so adherence to treatment is one of the crucial variables of effective ART programs. A continuous supply chain for drug access, tolerable and convenient treatment regimens, and counseling efforts can enhance adherence to ART (and ultimately provide a normal life expectancy including improving quality of life). It is expected that with the 2009 WHO ART guidelines, tolerability and convenience of the initial regimen will improve by withdrawing stavudine from the recommended list of nucleosides (WHO, 2009a, 2009b). Earlier initiation of treatment is another variable as it confers the potential benefits of reducing the mortality associated with treatment of late stage disease, diminishing transmission including transmission from mother-to-child in the peripartum and during breast-feeding, diminishing drug toxicity, and reducing treatment failure with its attendant development of drug resistance (Emery et al., 2008; Granich et al., 2010; Johansson et al., 2010; Kuhn et al., 2008; Kuhn, 2009; Lawn et al., 2008). Furthermore, treatment also confers other potential population health benefits such as reducing secondary transmission of HIV and TB (Corbett et al., 2003; Girardi et al., 2000; Granich et al., 2009; Lima et al., 2008; Montaner et al., 2006; von Linstow et al., 2010; Wood et al., 2009).

HIV drug resistance in treated patients is a measure of regimen efficacy and patient adherence; HIV drug resistance in treatment naïve patients is a measure of transmitted drug resistance. Consequently, monitoring for HIV drug resistance is important in order to assess program efficacy and future challenges with regard to different treatment regimens, maintaining a supply chain for drug access, providing care and counseling, and monitoring of treatment and its outcomes (WHO, 2006b). Under PEPFAR's laboratory program, PEPFAR's investments have provided support for the monitoring of drug resistance, which included "establishing HIV drug resistance testing capacity" and training of people from PEPFAR countries "on monitoring the emergence of drug resistance mutations in antiretroviral drug treated populations" (OGAC, 2009c, p. 128).

## Objective and Scope

The IOM evaluation of treatment programs under PEPFAR will assess the effects of these programs on long-term outcomes such as retention of people on treatment and increasing coverage and quality of services, as well as PEPFAR's contribution to improving the health of individuals and decreasing population level mortality due to HIV/AIDS.

This will include consideration of some health systems components. PEPFAR treatment programs, for purposes of budgeting and performance targets, include activities that directly or indirectly support the provision of ART. This includes the training of clinicians and other providers, clinical examinations, clinical monitoring, related laboratory services, and community-adherence activities—as well as procurement and in-freight delivery of ARV drugs (OGAC, 2009e). Like ARV drug procurement, all procurement for post-exposure prophylaxis for rape victims will be included under treatment activities. However, distribution, supply chain logistics, pharmaceutical management, and related systems-strengthening inputs do not fall under PEPFAR's treatment activities and will be assessed and evaluated under PEPFAR's health systems strengthening activities (see section 8 on Key Systems-Level Goals and Activities).

The evaluation of treatment programs will focus on PEPFAR's progress in achieving direct support of more than 4 million people on treatment (OGAC, 2009i)—the PEPFAR II programmatic target—and an assessment of the overall performance of treatment programs, including efforts to integrate with other health services and to address gender-specific aspects of HIV/AIDS treatment (see section 7 on Gender-Related Vulnerability and Risks). The committee might also find it necessary to consider some of the emerging issues identified by PEPFAR's TWG on Adult and Pediatric Treatment during the evaluation and assessment of treatment programs under PEPFAR. One of the main challenges that country programs face is continuing to scale up services for those in need while maintaining current numbers of people on treatment. Furthermore, according to PEPFAR's reauthorization, countries need to provide care and treatment services to HIV-infected children in proportion to the pediatric HIV burden in each country.[22] Its stated treatment and care goals for children in relation to allocation of funds across all treatment service categories over time may be valuable metrics for program "sustainability."

---

[22] *Supra.,* note 6 at §301(a)(2), 22 U.S.C. §2151b-2(b)(1)(A)(v).

Although the 2009 WHO guidelines on ART for adults, adolescents, and pregnant women substantially expand the population for whom treatment is indicated, PEPFAR's new Five-Year Strategy indicates that priority for access will focus on increasing access primarily within the "sickest," pregnant women, and patients with HIV and TB co-infection (OGAC, 2009i) (see Box 3). How to address treatment needs for the many eligible patients who may remain untreated is an important challenge. The evaluation committee can learn from the findings of detailed scholarly evaluations conducted by local researchers and the scientific communities of the partner countries related to overall access to treatment—conducted as a consequence of specific in-country decisions made and intended for future country leadership to learn from their historic experiences. Further, many challenges remain in the pediatric population, including issues with early identification and diagnosis and low access of ART in children less than 2 years old. This is compounded especially by inadequate funding for pediatric treatment—in several countries, UNITAID[23] and the Clinton Foundation are the sole purchasers of ART formulations and 2nd regimes for children, EID commodities, cotrimoxazole (CTX), and other drugs for opportunistic infections (OIs) (OGAC, 2009c; UNITAID-CHAI, 2010). UNICEF and UNAIDS have determined that about $6 billion of the $25 billion, needed by 2010 to enable countries to reach universal access goals,[24] is required to attain the universal goals specific to women and children (UNICEF, 2009). In 2010–2011, UNITAID and the Clinton Foundation will deliver the last shipment of some of these commodities; therefore, countries will need to make up for the gap (OGAC, 2009c). Since the United States alone cannot sustain ART for the millions of PLWHA, PEPFAR's focus under its new strategy is to support countries in discussing what resources are needed to respond to the HIV/AIDS epidemic, how to prioritize the large unmet need for treatment of adults, adolescents, and children, and how to identify resources for the gap—PEPFAR plans to support these efforts in a five-year plan through partnership frameworks with partner countries.

---

[23] UNITAID is an international facility dedicated to purchasing drugs for HIV/AIDS, malaria, and tuberculosis, primarily for people in low-income countries. UNITAID leverages its funds, received through airline ticket taxes or regular multi-year budget contributions from member countries, to reduce the price of quality diagnostics and medicines as well as to accelerate the development and availability of these products in low- and middle-income countries (UNITAID, 2010).

[24] At the United Nations General Assembly High-Level Meeting on AIDS in 2006, countries committed to work toward "universal access to comprehensive [HIV] prevention programmes, treatment, care and support by 2010" (United Nations General Assembly, 2006, p. 3).

---

**BOX 3**
**Areas of Emphasis in PEPFAR II's New Five-Year Strategy for Treatment**

- In partnership with country governments, PEPFAR is continuing the scale up of treatment to directly support more than 4 million people in its next phase.
- PEPFAR is working with countries to reach a threshold of 85 percent ARV prophylaxis or treatment of pregnant women found to be HIV-infected, in order to optimize maternal health and maximize HIV-free infant survival.
- In generalized epidemics, PEPFAR is working to reach a target of 65 percent early infant diagnosis, and support treatment for pediatric populations at a level commensurate with their representation in a larger country epidemic.
- Through country- and global-level efforts, PEPFAR is creating increased sustainability and capacity in treatment efforts and supporting countries in mobilizing and coordinating resources from multiple donors.
- PEPFAR is working with countries and international partners to expand identification and implementation of efficiencies in treatment, while ensuring continued expansion of measures to maintain adherence, quality, and retention in care.
- As part of the U.S. Global Health Initiative, PEPFAR is integrating its treatment programs with prevention and care portfolios, other health programs, and larger development efforts.

SOURCE: OGAC (2009i).

---

**Program Impact Pathway**

The evaluation approach for those activities under PEPFAR specific to adult and pediatric treatment will follow the impact pathway framework (see Figures 10 and 11). This approach is intended to illustrate how PEPFAR's investments and other laboratory commodities (inputs) for the delivery of ART services increase availability of ARVs and access to treatment interventions (outputs). Subsequently, the coverage of those in need of and eligible for treatment and the delivery of quality treatment services for HIV patients (outcomes) are expected to ultimately improve health of individuals and decrease population-level mortality (impacts). Time is required for the effects of the PEPFAR program on outcomes for a chronic disease like HIV/AIDS to become apparent and, more importantly for this evaluation, to accrue the systematic collection of valid and relevant data. Given the timely availability of quality data, the committee has developed examples of illustrative questions that it could address during the evaluation of PEPFAR. The committee developed a separate impact pathway for evaluating pediatric treatment considering the differences with adult treatment, including different points of entry for pediatric treatment services and socio-cultural barriers associated with the effective delivery of pediatric treatment by clinicians and non-clinicians, as well as the availability of drug formulations for children or appropriate use of adult preparations when substitutions are necessary (see Figure 11).

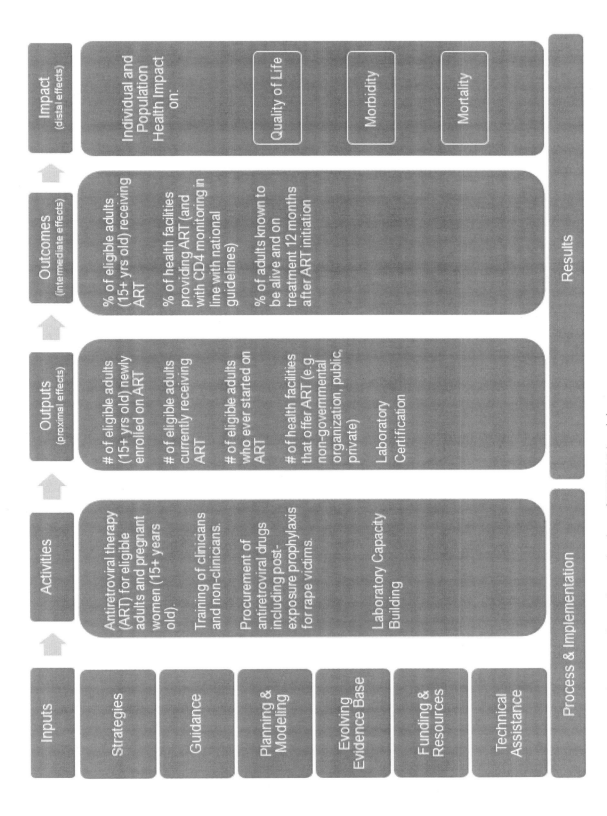

**FIGURE 10** Program impact pathway for evaluation of PEPFAR's adult treatment program.
NOTE: CD4 = cluster of differentiation 4.

86

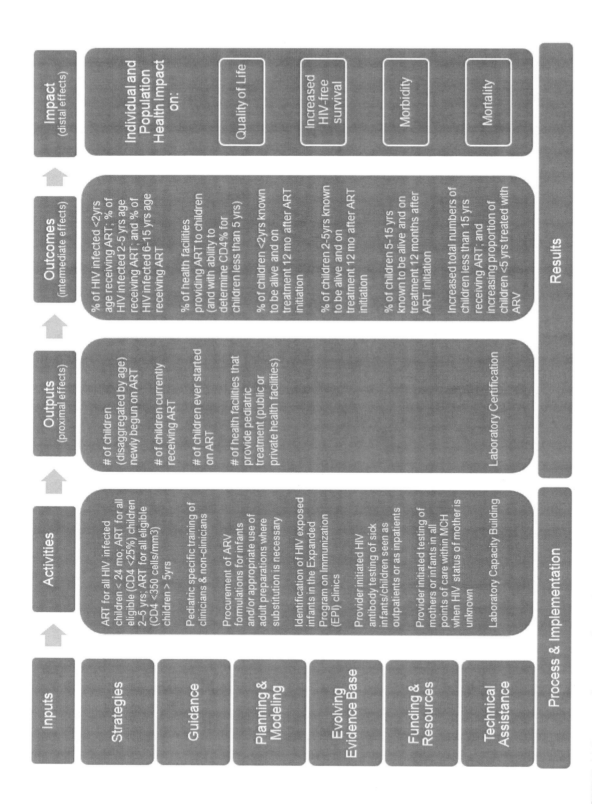

**FIGURE 11** Program impact pathway for evaluation of PEPFAR's pediatric treatment programs.
NOTES: ARV = antiretroviral drugs, ART = antiretroviral therapy, CD4 = cluster of differentiation 4, MCH = maternal and child health, mo = months old, yrs = years old.

## Illustrative Questions

Most of the limitations in evaluating the impact of treatment programs under PEPFAR and assessing their performance have to do with the fact that all the essential indicators gathered by OGAC from all partners are aggregated and limited. Age disaggregation is exceedingly important, especially to assess PEPFAR's performance in treating infants under 2 years old since ART, about one-third of HIV-infected infants will die by age 1 year and 50 percent by age 2 years (Newell et al., 2004). Meaningful data disaggregation will occur at the country level and, if available, are probably accessible through multilateral organizations such as UNAIDS and UNICEF, but without attribution to specific donors—these data will have to be requested. DHS and Multiple Indicator Cluster Survey (MICS data) will also need to be accessed in order to provide country context.

The following are examples of illustrative questions that the committee could address. These questions are intended to contribute to addressing part A, item ii and part B, items i and iv of the areas for consideration in the congressional mandate.[25]

*Is treatment funding (solo and joint PEPFAR and Global Fund) and provision of services being efficiently (equitably) distributed among countries, contractors, and implementers?*

*What is the number and proportion of adults and children with advanced HIV infection (i.e., CD4 <200 for adults) currently receiving ART?*

*What is the number and proportion of adults and children receiving treatment according to the updated WHO guidelines (i.e., all newborns, adults <350, all pregnant women)?*

*To what extent does the current methodology adequately or appropriately determine PEPFAR and Global Fund overlap in numbers?*

*What is the financial sustainability of existing and expanded coverage with treatment services, specifically ART? To what extent do PEPFAR activities or PEPFAR/Global Fund joint activities assist countries in determining and projecting costs for existing and expanded coverage with treatment services including ART?*

*To what extent are CD4 measurements being utilized to initiate treatment and monitor treatment?*

PEPFAR's NGO sub-partners, especially the Track 1.0 partners for treatment and care as well as the Presidential initiative for PMTCT that pre-dates PEPFAR I (but was subsequently subsumed within PEPFAR), have longitudinal reporting for as long as 10 years, and the ability to disaggregate by facility, as well as by many other parameters. Longitudinal, individual patient

---

[25] (A)(ii) an evaluation of the impact on health of prevention, treatment, and care efforts that are supported by United States funding, including multilateral and bilateral programs involving joint operations
(B)(i) an assessment of progress toward prevention, treatment, and care targets
(B)(iv) an evaluation of the impact of treatment and care programs on 5-year survival rates, drug adherence, and the emergence of drug resistance

data are available only from very few of sub-partners, but do include large numbers of people. The most detailed information will therefore represent specific facilities in selected countries.

> *What are the rates of drug resistance in treated and naïve populations? How are these data used for policymaking decisions about selection of treatment regimens?*

PEPFFAR supports the WHO's strategy on HIV drug resistance surveillance and monitoring, and has provided support to build drug resistance testing capacity in PEPFAR countries (OGAC, 2009c). Globally, the WHO HIV drug resistance threshold survey method is being implemented in resource-limited countries to determine transmitted drug resistance levels as part of the surveillance of transmitted HIV drug resistance. The results of these surveys are published in scientific journals. The committee will seek to collect these published papers in order to assess the effects of treatment programs on the emergence of drug resistance.

> *What percent of adults, children, and pregnant women who initiated ART are alive and on treatment at 1 year and annually thereafter?*

Although treatment adherence is considered essential to successful therapy as well as to extending regimens and reducing medication and hospitalization costs, none of the OGAC indicators measure it. However, in the provision of treatment at the facility, district, and sub-partner levels, adherence has been monitored because it is necessary for the delivery of therapy. Some of the sub-partners, interested in quality of care, have routinely monitored adherence (albeit with multiple and not always standardized or validated definitions). Monitoring is usually done via return visits, pill counts, clinical assessment, and self-report. The proportion of the population on second-line regimens is another measure, although without genotyping/phenotyping it is not always clear whether regimen failure is due to non-adherence. Learning what the individual countries require will guide the committee's effort to answer questions on adherence.

Currently, assessing the impact of ART programs on mortality at the population level will be limited due to the lack of vital statistical data or the delay in generating vital statistics in many of the PEPFAR countries. Many low- and middle-income countries have inadequate vital or civil registration systems and where the systems exist, they are usually not comprehensive and the cause of death is misreported or underreported (WHO et al., 2009). "Surveys conducted sometimes use verbal autopsies to retrospectively assess HIV-attributable mortality in a population; however, this approach often lacks baseline data for assessing how access to ART affects HIV-related mortality. Some countries have also counted burials of deceased people in the age group of 15–49 years" (WHO et al., 2009). Therefore, although an evaluation of the impact of treatment on 5-year survival of HIV-infected adults and children receiving ART has been requested in the congressional mandate, any survival data will be limited and mortality data greater than one- to two-year survival will not be available for most PEPFAR treatment programs.

## SECTION 5: CARE AND SUPPORT SERVICES

Care and support services are an important component of PEPFAR and other donor programs for HIV/AIDS. PEPFAR defines care and support services as "the wide range of services other than ART offered to people living with HIV/AIDS (PLWHA) and other affected persons, such as family members" (OGAC, 2009a, p. 16). During FY2009, PEPFAR directly supported care and support for nearly 11 million people affected by HIV/AIDS, including 7 million HIV-infected individuals and approximately 4 million orphans and vulnerable children (OGAC, 2010). Care and support includes clinical, psychological, social, spiritual, and preventive services that may be provided in facility-, community-, or home-based settings. The Lantos–Hyde Act of 2008 charges PEPFAR II to support care for 12 million people infected with or affected by HIV/AIDS (including 5 million children orphaned or made otherwise vulnerable by HIV/AIDS), "with an emphasis on promoting a comprehensive, coordinated system of services to be integrated throughout the continuum of care."[26] Efforts to integrate care and support services with broader health and development programs, such as voluntary family planning and reproductive health services, are a key component of PEPFAR II (OGAC, 2009g). As outlined in the new Five-Year Strategy (2009–2013), PEPFAR has adopted a "woman- and girl-centered approach" to delivering services, which "takes into account the realities of women's and girls' lives as shaped by gender norms, service availability, and larger structural factors," and is working to ensure that other marginalized populations have equal access to services (OGAC, 2009h, p. 6, 2009i).

### Components of PEPFAR Care and Support Services

The latest PEPFAR-issued guidance for care and support services, "Guidance for United States Government In-Country Staff and Implementing Partners for a Preventive Care Package for Adults," was released in 2006 and describes a menu of preventive care services for adults (OGAC, 2006b). A similar menu of services for children (0–14 years) was also released in 2006 and is described in the Child and Adolescent Well-Being section of this report. These preventive care services (see Figure 12) are intended to promote health and quality of life for PLWHA, slow the progression of AIDS, and reduce HIV-related complications and mortality. The preventive care services for adults include five of the thirteen interventions considered essential by WHO for adults and adolescents living with HIV in resource-limited settings (five additional interventions are delivered through PEPFAR prevention and treatment services) (OGAC, 2006b; WHO, 2008).

---

[26] *Supra.*, note 6 at §101(a), 22 U.S.C. §7611(a)(4)(C).

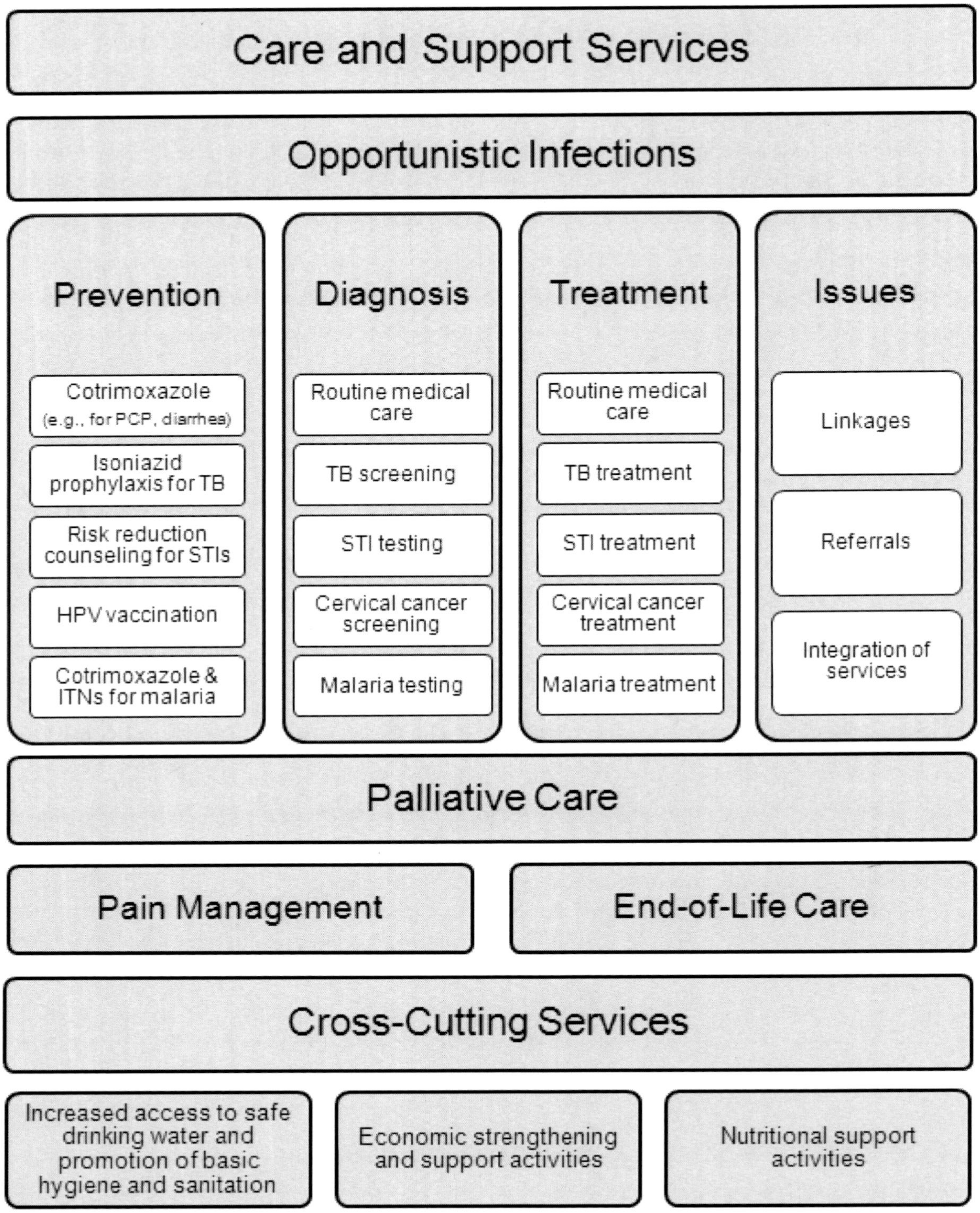

**FIGURE 12** PEPFAR care and support services.
NOTES: HPV = human papillomavirus; ITNs = insecticide-treated nets; PCP = *Pneumocystis jiroveci* pneumonia; STI = sexually transmitted infections; TB = tuberculosis.

Although the type of interventions in a preventive care menu will differ by region or country according to the capacity of implementing partners, some recommended components include:

*Screening, Prophylaxis, and Treatment for Tuberculosis*

TB and HIV co-infection is very common and has devastating consequences for PLWHA. HIV infection increases the risk of TB 10-fold, and in sub-Saharan Africa and Asia, TB is the leading cause of death for PLWHA (WHO, 2008). WHO guidelines recommend counseling (education) and regular TB screening for all PLWHA, and preventive therapy (isoniazid) for HIV-infected patients with latent TB (WHO, 2008). In order to identify people who have HIV infection, PEPFAR efforts have focused on the scale-up of same-day HIV testing at TB clinics. However, even in countries where this scale-up has been effective, a large number of TB patients identified as HIV-positive are lost to follow up after referrals to HIV/AIDS care and treatment programs, and efforts to screen, diagnosis, and treat all HIV patients for TB have been less successful (OGAC, 2009c). Further, lack of laboratory capacity has hindered efforts to scale up isoniazid preventive therapy for PLWHA with latent TB infection, as many countries lack the ability to rule out active TB, a prerequisite for isoniazid prophylaxis (OGAC, 2009c). The new Five-Year Strategy commits PEPFAR to scale up efforts to screen, diagnose, and if necessary, treat all HIV patients for TB, while expanding linkages and referrals to ensure that all TB patients are tested for HIV and if positive, referred to treatment (OGAC, 2009g, 2009h).

*Prophylactic Drugs for Opportunistic Infections*

CTX is a broad-spectrum antimicrobial agent that prevents *Pneumocystis jiroveci* pneumonia (formerly *Pneumocystis carinii* pneumonia), toxoplasmosis, and malaria (WHO, 2006a). WHO recommends that all adults with HIV receive CTX prophylaxis indefinitely as a cost-effective method to significantly reduce morbidity and mortality, but country-level policies vary according to the burden of HIV and other diseases, as well as the capacity and infrastructure of health systems (WHO, 2008). WHO also recommends that all infants born to HIV-infected mothers receive CTX (WHO, 2006a). Cryptococcal disease is common and often treatable in PLWHA, but many countries lack the infrastructure and human capacity for diagnosis (OGAC, 2009c; WHO, 2008). PEPFAR has provided limited training and laboratory capacity building for diagnosis, but without early recognition, mortality from cryptococcal disease is high (OGAC, 2009c). Where cryptococcal disease is common and diagnostic capacity exists, WHO recommends consideration of antifungal prophylaxis (fluconazole or itraconazole) for severely immunocompromised PLWHA (WHO, 2008). Currently, there is limited availability of antifungal prophylaxis, but PEPFAR is working with its Supply Chain Management System and Pfizer, which runs a fluconazole donation program, to increase access to drugs for treatment and prevention (OGAC, 2009c).

*Improved Screening and Treatment of Opportunistic Infections (including Cervical Cancer)*

Screening and diagnosis of OIs may be limited by human and laboratory capacity in many countries. Cervical cancer is almost always caused by certain types of human papilloma virus. Cancer-causing strains of human papilloma virus are common in women with HIV and increase the risk of cervical cancer (OGAC, 2009c). WHO recommends that where available, women with HIV should be screened for cervical cancer annually (WHO, 2008). As part of a comprehensive approach to OIs, PEPFAR is currently supporting "pilot programs which provide screening and treatment to prevent cervical cancer in HIV-positive women" (OGAC, 2009a, p. 55). These pilot programs are using the "see and treat" approach, which includes visual inspection with acetic acid, visual inspection with Lugol's iodine, and direct visual inspection (Kaur and Singh, 2010).

*Increased Access to Safe Drinking Water to Prevent Waterborne Illnesses and the Promotion of Basic Hygiene and Sanitation to Reduce Exposure to Pathogens*

In many developing countries, poor infrastructure and lack of safe management of human waste increase the risk of waterborne and enteric pathogens, many of which cause diarrhea (WHO, 2008). Diarrhea affects 90 percent of PLWHA, and interventions to improve water, sanitation, and hygiene, such as provision of safe water storage vessels and education regarding hand-washing, can greatly reduce diarrhea-related morbidity (OGAC, 2009c). The latest USG "Framework for Addressing Water Challenges in the Developing World," which guides USAID and DoS efforts, encourages the incorporation of these interventions into all HIV/AIDS programs (USAID and DoS, 2009). PEPFAR's preventive care package also includes water purification systems, which in combination with other health interventions, may keep PLWHA healthy and delay the need for treatment (OGAC, 2009a).

*Prevention of Malaria*

WHO recommends the integration of malaria and HIV services with a particular focus on prevention (WHO, 2008). As previously mentioned, CTX may reduce malaria-related morbidity and mortality in PLWHA. Insecticide-treated nets (ITNs), when used properly and regularly, are cost-effective and greatly reduce exposure to malaria infection. WHO also recommends intermittent preventive therapy (IPTp), which can reduce the risk of malaria and its consequences, for HIV-positive pregnant women who are not taking CTX (WHO, 2008). The President's Malaria Initiative (PMI) is a USG interagency initiative to reduce malaria in 15 focus countries, 9 of which have significant PEPFAR programs (PMI, 2009). PMI is working to expand coverage of effective malaria prevention and treatment interventions, including ITNs, indoor residual spraying with insecticides, IPTp, and artemisinin-based combination therapy (PMI, 2009). PEPFAR routinely links to PMI, and their efforts overlap in ITN distribution and education programs as well as coordination of lab services (OGAC, 2009a).

*Food and Nutrition Support Services*

HIV infection may cause or intensify malnutrition by reducing appetites, increasing energy needs, and impairing nutrient absorption in PLWHA (OGAC, 2009c). Proper nutrition supports the immune system, preventing OIs. Nutritional and micronutrient supplementation may reduce HIV-related morbidity and mortality and improve outcomes for patients on ART (OGAC, 2009i). Through its Food by Prescription programs, PEPFAR targets clinically malnourished children and adults with HIV infection, pregnant and lactating women and their infants in PMTCT programs, and orphans and other vulnerable children (regardless of HIV status) for food and nutrition care and support, including nutrition assessment and counseling services, specialized food products, and micronutrient supplementation (OGAC, 2009c). Although PEPFAR does not support direct food distribution to families, the new Five-Year Strategy emphasizes linkages and referrals of those in need to the new USG Global Hunger and Food Security Initiative, Title II programs, and other initiatives such as the World Food Program (OGAC, 2009c, 2009g).

*Health, Dignity, and Prevention Programming for PLHWA and Their Families*

Health, Dignity, and Prevention programming includes efforts related to health promotion and education, reducing stigma for PLWHA, and preventing HIV transmission from infected to non-infected people. The components of the preventive care package recommended by PEPFAR address health promotion, and prevention efforts are discussed in this report's prevention section. PEPFAR is working with country governments to develop "policies that address the drivers of the epidemic in country and provide equitable access to quality services for marginalized populations" and expanding "linkages to multiple primary and specialty health services" which "increases community-level access to quality care and reduces the stigma associated with HIV" (OGAC, 2009i, pp. 15, 27).

*Palliative Care, Including Management of Pain and Other Symptoms*

PEPFAR defines palliative care as an "holistic approach to providing services that includes a focus on pain and symptom management and on improving quality of life," which is consistent with the WHO definition (OGAC, 2009c, p. 25). Palliative care, including pain management and end-of-life care, enables PLWHA to lead happier, more productive lives and reduces the burden of care on families. In many countries, restrictive policy environments prohibit effective pain management programs, and access to strong pain medications such as opioids is limited (OGAC, 2009i). Up to 80 percent of those with advanced HIV infection experience pain, and pain management programs can greatly improve quality of life for PLWHA (OGAC, 2009c). PEPFAR's new strategy calls for continued efforts to "support policy changes that ensure pain management is included both in guidelines and actual clinical services for PLWHAs," as well as increased efforts to "strengthen commodity systems, train providers, and expand access to opioids for pain management" (OGAC, 2009i, p. 19).

*Economic Strengthening and Support Activities*

Recognizing that a lack of economic assets increases vulnerability to HIV infection, PEPFAR supports economic strengthening and support activities that "supply, protect, or grow physical, natural, financial, human, and social assets" (OGAC, 2009h, p. 17). These activities may include microfinance and microcredit programs to expand access to financial services, vocational training to offer alternatives to transactional sex, and income-generating activities, such as communal gardens (that may also provide food).

**Objective and Scope**

With regard to care and support services, the committee is charged to evaluate the impact on health of care efforts supported by USG funding and assess progress toward care targets. Complicating this task, country-level guidelines for ART eligibility differ and make program-wide comparisons difficult. The committee is also charged to evaluate impact of care programs on 5-year survival rates among people not yet eligible for ARV treatment. Data on 5-year survival rates is very limited for any population; unless these data are being collected and can be accessed, it will not be possible to assess PEPFAR's impact on 5-year survival rates among people not yet eligible for ART.

## Program Impact Pathway

To assess whether PEPFAR has achieved targets regarding care and support services, the committee will examine PEPFAR's care and support activities and use output and outcome indicators (e.g., number of people accessing care services, percent of HIV-positive patients provided CTX prophylaxis) where available. To evaluate the impact of care services on health, the committee will use a combination of output and outcome indicators to determine the extent of delivery of PEPFAR-funded services in-country. Figure 13 depicts the committee's understanding of some of PEPFAR's care and support activities and some potential outputs and outcomes to be measured during the evaluation.

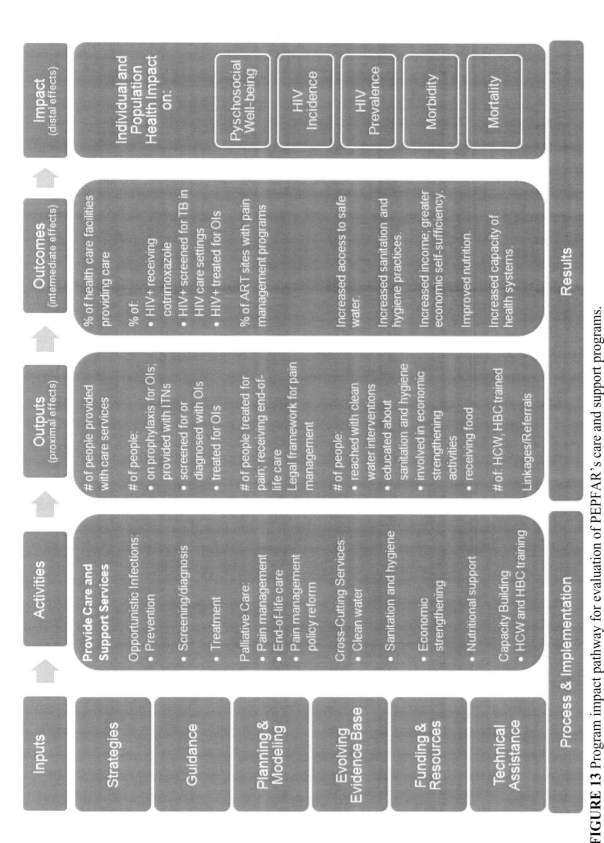

**FIGURE 13** Program impact pathway for evaluation of PEPFAR's care and support programs.
NOTES: ART = antiretroviral therapy; HBC = home-based care workers; HCW = heath care workers; ITNs = insecticide-treated nets; OIs = opportunistic infections; TB = tuberculosis.

**Illustrative Questions**

Care is composed of multiple components, and the complexities of measurement are increased by what is included or has changed over time during PEPFAR (i.e., 14 of the essential PEPFAR indicators of care have changed significantly, have been dropped, or are new).[27] The lack of consistently measured data may result in data gaps that limit the possibility of examining longitudinal trends. Given the timely availability of quality data, the following are examples of illustrative questions that the committee could address. These questions are intended to contribute to addressing part A, item ii and part B, items i and iv of the areas for consideration in the congressional mandate.[28]

*What populations are accessing care and support services?*

The number and types of populations accessing care will be measured through quantitative analysis of PEPFAR indicators. Aggregated data reported to OGAC provide limited insight about the types of populations accessing care, so the committee will seek disaggregated data from other sources. To reflect PEPFAR's new women- and girl-centered approach to delivering services and the emphasis on equity across marginalized populations, the committee will seek data disaggregated by sex and population type (IDUs, MSM, etc.). Measurement of the number of people receiving care services is complicated by the potential of "double counting" (people accessing more than one service may be counted more than once).

*What is the access to prophylaxis for, diagnosis of, and treatment of OIs? How has treatment for TB been maximized with jointly operated activities between PEPFAR and the Global Fund? How has coverage expanded as result of joint efforts? What has been the effect on grantee performance to improve access?*

There are several PEPFAR indicators that measure the number and percentage of HIV-positive patients receiving CTX, isoniazid preventive therapy, and TB screening and treatment (OGAC, 2009d). In addition to the aggregated data reported to OGAC, the committee will seek additional data sources to provide information regarding testing and treatment for malaria and sexually transmitted infections, treatment for pneumonia and diarrhea, vaccinations for human papilloma virus, and more. The committee will also seek information regarding human and laboratory capacity building to increase diagnostic capabilities for OIs.

*How is PEPFAR supporting access to and distribution of ITNs? How is this measured?*

There are no PEPFAR indicators regarding ITNs. The committee will seek information from PMI or implementing NGOs or contractors that receive PEPFAR funding to distribute ITNs.

---

[27] Essential indicators are those for which OGAC requires PEPFAR Country Teams to track data to monitor PEPFAR's progress (OGAC, 2009d).

[28] (A)(ii) an evaluation of the impact on health of prevention, treatment, and care efforts that are supported by United States funding, including multilateral and bilateral programs involving joint operations

(B)(i) an assessment of progress toward prevention, treatment, and care targets

(B)(iv) an evaluation of the impact of treatment and care programs on 5-year survival rates, drug adherence, and the emergence of drug resistance

*How is PEPFAR supporting access to safe drinking water, basic hygiene, and sanitation? How is this measured? Is there any discernible effect of this access for improved health or a decrease in OIs diagnosed and needing treatment?*

There are no PEPFAR indicators regarding safe drinking water, basic hygiene, and sanitation. The committee will seek data and information regarding access to safe water, ideally multi-year data to examine trends, from countries, implementing agencies, partners, sub-partners, and international stakeholders. Some data may be available from implementing NGOs or contractors that receive PEPFAR funding to conduct activities regarding basic hygiene and sanitation.

*How is PEPFAR incorporating palliative care or pain management into care services? What is the proportion of need compared to availability of services, particularly analgesics and opioids? Are PEPFAR teams following WHO guidelines for provision of analgesics including opioids?*

PEPFAR indicators measure the percentage of ART sites that have pain management programs and the progress toward incorporating pain management into national HIV/AIDS strategies, but the committee will seek additional information from other sources. The committee will also seek information from the Palliative Care TWG at OGAC about proposed activities for and guidance to Country Teams to develop or change policies in the country related to drug procurement, drug security, and scope of practice for dispensing drugs to patients.

*What economic support and strengthening activities does PEPFAR support? How is this measured?*

There is one PEPFAR indicator that measures the number of eligible adults and children provided with economic support or strengthening services, but the committee will need to seek additional information regarding the types of economic support and strengthening activities and their effectiveness from other sources.

*Who is receiving therapeutic or supplementary food and through what activities? Is there a discernible effect on ART adherence or mortality?*

PEPFAR indicators measure the number of people receiving food or nutrition services and the percent of HIV-positive clinically malnourished patients receiving food. The committee will use aggregated data reported to OGAC and seek disaggregated data from organizations and initiatives to which PEPFAR links or refers HIV-positive patients for nutritional support.

## SECTION 6: CHILD AND ADOLESCENT WELL-BEING

The HIV/AIDS pandemic has produced devastating effects on the lives of millions of children and adolescents[29] worldwide endangering their development, life course, and survival. When HIV affects parents and other adult caregivers, it destroys their families and deprives them of care and protection by weakening communities and social support networks, welfare systems, and economies. Moreover, millions of children and adolescents are currently directly affected due to infection with HIV. In 2008, children under 15 years of age were estimated to be nearly 16 percent of incident cases, and the number of children under 15 years of age living with HIV/AIDS worldwide was approximately two million, with an additional number of adolescents among the 31 million adults (age 15 and over) living with the disease (UNAIDS and WHO, 2009). In 2007, the number of children and adolescents aged 0–17 years old who have lost one or both parents as a result of the AIDS epidemic[30] was estimated to be approximately 15 million worldwide—in sub-Saharan Africa alone, the number was estimated to be approximately 12 million children (UNAIDS, 2008). Combining the needs of children and adolescents infected with HIV with the needs of orphans, as well as other children and adolescents made vulnerable due to HIV/AIDS, gives a full perspective on the burden of the epidemic in these populations. Therefore, understanding the needs of all children and adolescents affected and made vulnerable by HIV/AIDS is a vital step in the response to the HIV/AIDS pandemic (JLICA, 2009).

In addition to the need for access to HIV/AIDS services, there are also other critical developmental and societal factors influencing the health and psychosocial well-being of children and adolescents affected by HIV/AIDS. For example, many children and adolescents with sick and dying parents have to become the breadwinners and primary caregivers of their households (Cluver et al., 2007). When a parent dies, some of the effects related to the grieving process, as well as the deprivation and life changes that occur because of this loss, might affect the health and well-being of the lost parent's children. Parental loss might result in trauma, relocation, loss of a breadwinner, residence in poorer households, and living with less closely related caregivers, which can lead to other effects including poorer access to adequate nutrition, shelter, and health care, and lack of educational support. These are all mediating factors of psychosocial well-being (Cluver and Orkin, 2009; Nyamukapa et al., 2008). Children and adolescents, in settings where HIV is highly stigmatized, have to cope with higher levels of psychosocial stressors associated with the loss of a parent due to HIV/AIDS than both children orphaned by other causes and non-orphaned children (Cluver and Gardner, 2007; Cluver and Orkin, 2009). Children and adolescents living within communities that experience a high HIV

---

[29] The committee uses "children and adolescents" as a general term without a specific age definition, recognizing that the ages used to categorize children and adolescents vary by data source and organization. In particular, the age categories vary for terms like adolescents, youth, and young people. For example, adolescents are defined by WHO as young men and women 10–19 years of age and young people refers to men and women 10–24 years of age (WHO, 1999, 2006c). United Nations defines youth as men and women 15–24 years of age and young people refers to men and women 10–24 years of age (WHO, 1999, 2006c). Within PEPFAR, defined age ranges vary by programmatic area. Throughout this section, the specific age ranges used by PEPFAR or by the cited data source are indicated whenever feasible.

[30] In 2001, a consensus was reached among members of the UNAIDS Reference Group on Estimates Modelling and Projection, and international researchers on the definition of orphans due to HIV/AIDS. An "AIDS orphan" was defined as a child who has at least one parent who has died due to AIDS and a dual (or double) "AIDS orphan" as a child whose mother and father have both died, at least one due to AIDS (UNAIDS Reference Group on Estimates Modelling and Projections, 2002).

burden are at a greater risk of these forms of vulnerabilities, and are at a greater risk of physical and sexual abuse, sexual exploitation, homelessness, and exposure to HIV (UNAIDS et al., 2002, 2004).

In addition to younger children, the vulnerabilities of youth between the ages of 15–24 years have been recognized by the international community (UNGASS, 2001; WHO et al., 1997). This developmental period is an important transition period, and youth are vulnerable due to age-specific changes that are physical (their physical and cognitive abilities), psychological (how they think about themselves), and social (their relationships and roles, expectations, economic security, and citizenship). These changes have implications for how they understand information and what influences them, how they think about the future and make decisions in the present, and how they perceive risk and their sexual behavior (Dick, 2009).

In 2007, an estimated 45 percent of incident cases in people aged 15 years and older were found among youth aged 15–24 years. Overall, in 2008, a total of approximately 5 million youth aged 15–24 years were living with HIV in low- and middle-income countries (UNICEF, 2009), and in sub-Saharan Africa, youth, and in particular young women, are disproportionately vulnerable and therefore at greater risk of HIV infection (Gouws et al., 2008; Napierala-Mavedzenge et al., 2010; UNAIDS and WHO, 2009; UNICEF, 2009). Beyond biological susceptibility to HIV, socio-cultural factors that contribute to the vulnerability of young women to sexually transmitted HIV infection include entrenched gender roles, unbalanced power relations, sexual violence (such as coerced sex), unsafe sex with older men, and a lack of skills and information about how to protect themselves and access services (UNAIDS, 2009a) (see section on Gender-Related Vulnerability and Risk).

The International Convention on the Rights of the Child,[31] guides the international community's efforts to protect the rights of children under the age of 18 years to survival, development, and access to health services, including a focus on reversing the HIV epidemic in children and mitigating its negative effects on their health and well-being through the MDGs, the UNGASS on HIV/AIDS, and the UNGASS on Children (UNICEF, 2007). The progress of countries in achieving the standards and goals outlined in these documents is monitored by the Committee on the Rights of the Child (CRC), primarily through country reports that may provide valuable information for this evaluation on the environment in which PEPFAR's efforts to improve child and adolescent well-being are operating within a specific country or region.

Efforts by multilateral and bilateral stakeholders to support policy on orphans and vulnerable children and adolescents affected by HIV/AIDS have resulted in the development of the "Framework for the Protection, Care, and Support of Orphans and Vulnerable Children Living in a World with HIV and AIDS," which PEPFAR has adopted (IOM, 2007). This framework document lays out five key strategies to improve the well-being of children: (1) strengthening the capacity of families, (2) mobilizing and supporting community-based responses, (3) ensuring access for orphans and vulnerable children to essential services, (4) ensuring that governments protect the most vulnerable children through improved policy and

---

[31] The Convention on the Rights of the Child is the first legally binding international instrument to incorporate the full range of civil, cultural, economic, political, and social rights of children. The Convention gives UNICEF the responsibility of promoting the rights of children by supporting the Committee on the Rights of the Child (CRC). As the oversight body, the CRC monitors the progress of State Parties in setting and meeting the standards outlined in the Convention. UNICEF provides technical assistance to governments on the implementation of the Convention and the development of implementing reports, which are required to be submitted by State Parties to the CRC 2 years after acceding to the Convention and every 5 years thereafter. The CRC convenes three times a year to review the States' reports (OHCHR, 2007; United Nations, 1990; United Nations Treaty Collection, 2010).

legislation, and (5) raising awareness at all levels through advocacy and social mobilization to create a supportive environment (UNAIDS et al., 2002, 2004; UNICEF, 2004).

## PEPFAR-Supported Interventions for Children and Adolescents

PEPFAR currently supports services for children and adolescents through its three main programmatic areas—prevention, care, and treatment. Additionally, in keeping with the "Framework for the Protection, Care, and Support of Orphans and Vulnerable Children Living in a World with HIV and AIDS," PEPFAR supports programs specifically identified for orphans and vulnerable children and adolescents (hereinafter referred to as OVC programs or programming[32]). In FY2009, PEPFAR supported care for 3,620,140 million children and adolescents through its OVC programming, and provided pediatric treatment for 201,500 individuals under 15 years of age (about 8 percent of the total number of people receiving ART with direct PEPFAR support) (OGAC, 2010). In addition, 273,100 individuals were trained or retained on the care and support of orphans and vulnerable children and adolescents (OGAC, 2010). Other PEPFAR-supported capacity building during this fiscal year to address the needs of children included the training or retaining of 62,100 healthcare workers on PMTCT services (including 15,597 PMTCT service facilities) (OGAC, 2010).

The Lantos–Hyde Act of 2008 underscores children and adolescent needs as part of the USG commitment of preventing 12,000,000 new HIV infections worldwide and increasing the number of individuals with HIV/AIDS receiving ART. In particular, it states that programs supported by PEPFAR need to "provide care and treatment services to children with HIV in proportion to their percentage within the HIV-infected population of a given partner country."[33] Additionally, PEPFAR II performance targets for the care and support of PLWHA include providing care and support for five million children and adolescents orphaned or made otherwise vulnerable by HIV/AIDS.[34] In order to achieve this target, the new Five-Year Strategy states that PEPFAR will continue to address child-development issues through child-focused programming that targets the full range of needs at different developmental stages (OGAC, 2006e, 2009i, p. 22) (see Box 4). Within the scope of care and support activities for PLWHA, the act directs that "at least 10 percent"[35] of PEPFAR funds supporting country activities for prevention, treatment, and care go to OVC programs in order to mitigate the impact of HIV/AIDS for millions of children and adolescents living in affected communities—an earmark that was preserved in the reauthorization legislation. In FY2009, these funds amounted to approximately $320 million,[36] with an additional $44 million provided in funding for pediatric care and support activities (OGAC, 2009f).

Finally, the Lantos–Hyde Act of 2008 also highlights a new emphasis on the transition to young adulthood. The reauthorization legislation states that PEPFAR's annual report to Congress will include a description of the strategies, goals, programs, and interventions that "address the needs and vulnerabilities of youth populations" and "expand access among young men and women to evidence-based HIV/AIDS health care services and HIV prevention programs."[37] To

---

[32] For the purpose of brevity, the acronym OVC will be used to describe programs targeting eligible children and adolescents under PEPFAR's programs for orphan and vulnerable children.

[33] *Supra.*, note 6 at §301(a)(2), 22 U.S.C. §2151b-2(b)(1)(A)(v).

[34] *Ibid.*, §301(a)(2), 22 U.S.C. §2151b-2(b)(1)(A)(iii).

[35] *Supra.*, note 1 at §403(b), 22 U.S.C. §7673(b).

[36] Approved funds in FY2009 for supporting OVC programs' activities found in PEPFAR operational plans.

[37] *Supra.*, note 6 at §301(a)(2), 22 U.S.C. §2151-b2(f)(2)(D)(ix).

reflect the new priorities in programming that address the age-specific needs and vulnerabilities of adolescents and young people in particular, PEPFAR II is committing through its new Five-Year Strategy to support countries in pursuing these objectives (see Box 4).

---

**BOX 4**
**Reauthorization Programming for Orphans and Vulnerable Children**

**Years 1–2:**
- Support countries to define, map, and plan a prioritized, multisectoral response to the needs of OVC populations and sub-populations within a country.
- Work with partner countries to identify gaps in capacity, including gaps in coordination among ministries overseeing education, food and nutrition, social welfare, and health.
- Establish training, mentoring, and technical assistance programs in partnership with governments in order to increase the number of professional staff in all agencies who can address cross-cutting OVC needs.
- Work with countries to increase support for family-based care by establishing and strengthening linkages between clinical and home- and community-based care.
- Scale up and ensure robust monitoring of existing high-impact OVC programs and support countries in developing, implementing, and evaluating innovative OVC pilot programming.
- Help countries ensure that policies for most-at-risk populations have adequate coverage and referrals for youth subpopulations.
- Support countries in developing a case management capability to assist the transition of young adults from OVC services into society and careers.

**Years 3–5:**
- Work with countries to engage in periodic and targeted surveys and other evaluations to determine impact of OVC programming.
- Ensure that countries have programs through which OVC can access livelihood development opportunities, including vocational training and microenterprise development training, to support themselves and their families.

SOURCE: OGAC (2009i).

---

*Prevention*

The Lantos–Hyde Act of 2008 emphasizes the need to intensify efforts to prevent HIV as a priority within the USG-supported response to the global HIV epidemic.[38] The majority of new incident cases in infants and young children occur from transmission in utero, during delivery, or post-partum as a result of breastfeeding (UNAIDS and WHO, 2009). In 2008, an estimated 1.4 million pregnant women living with HIV in low- and middle-income countries gave birth (WHO et al., 2009). PMTCT, also described previously in the section on Prevention, is an evidence-based prevention intervention that can reduce perinatal HIV transmission to approximately 2 percent if appropriately delivered under optimal circumstances (Cunningham et al., 2002;

---

[38] *Ibid.*, §4, 22 U.S.C. § 7603(3)(A).

Dorenbaum et al., 2002; Kuhn et al., 2008). UNAIDS estimated that 200,000 cumulative new HIV infections have been averted in the past 12 years through the provision of ARV drugs for prophylaxis to HIV-positive pregnant women (UNAIDS and WHO, 2009). Similar to other bilateral and multilateral stakeholders, such as the Global Fund, PEPFAR II strategic plans include expanding access to PMTCT services "as a mechanism to both prevent transmission of HIV to children and support expanded access to care and related services for pregnant women" (OGAC, 2009i, p. 9). PEPFAR II targets, aligned to follow the targets for PMTCT of the Declaration of Commitment on HIV/AIDS, commits to providing "at least 80 percent of the target population with access to counseling, testing, and treatment to prevent the transmission of HIV from mother-to-child."[39] In FY2009, PEPFAR reported that 509,800 HIV-positive pregnant women received ARV prophylaxis, and estimated approximately 96,862 infant HIV infections averted (OGAC, 2010).

In addition, PEPFAR supports other prevention interventions that are "medically accurate, age-appropriate, and targeted to the needs based upon behavior" (OGAC, 2009i, p. 12; PEPFAR, 2008b). PEPFAR's activities aimed at prevention of sexually transmitted HIV target at-risk youth (OGAC, 2009e), and PEPFAR is supporting prevention programming for young people (10–24 years old) (OGAC, 2009a). Country activities that support "efforts to expand HIV counseling and testing, which are entry points to care and treatment," also serve orphans and vulnerable children and adolescents (OGAC, 2009a, p. 52).

*Treatment*

PEPFAR also serves the needs of children and adolescents through its treatment programs including appropriate pediatric formulations for HIV-infected infants and eligible children (ages 0–14) (see section on Adult and Pediatric Treatment). In addition to improving clinical outcomes and increasing survival in HIV-infected children and adolescents on ART, overall population improvements in access to ART may also have benefits for children and adolescents. Recent studies suggest that improved availability and coverage of ART may reduce the number of children and adolescents who will be orphaned due to HIV in the next couple of years (Mermin et al., 2008; Stover et al., 2008; UNAIDS, 2008; UNAIDS and WHO, 2009). In the FY2009 report to Congress, PEPFAR estimated that the number of orphans averted through PEPFAR-supported treatment programs was approximately 1.6 million through September 30, 2008. However, the availability of data and methods for estimating the effects of ART in protecting children and adolescents from orphanhood continues to be a challenge as more information is gathered on ART coverage and the current needs of child and adolescent populations infected or affected by HIV/AIDS (UNAIDS Reference Group on Estimates Modelling and Projections, 2002, 2007).

*Care and Support*

PEPFAR commits to supporting comprehensive care interventions other than ART to meet the new targets of providing care and support for 12 million people infected with or affected by HIV/AIDS, including 5 million children and adolescents orphaned or made otherwise vulnerable by HIV/AIDS,[40] (see section on Care and Support Services). In addition to PEPFAR-

---

[39] *Ibid.*, §301(a)(2), 22 U.S.C. §2151b-2(b)(1)(A)(iv).
[40] *Ibid.*, §301(a)(2), 22 U.S.C. §2151b-2(b)(1)(A)(iii).

supported pediatric care and support activities described here, the specific OVC programs described later are also among the HIV/AIDS care interventions that PEPFAR supports (OGAC, 2006e, p. 3).

PEPFAR's "Guidance for United States Government In-Country Staff and Implementing Partners for a Preventive Care Package for Children Aged 0–14 Years Old Born to HIV-Infected Mothers - #1," which was released in April 2006, describes PEPFAR-supported activities for children born to HIV-infected mothers (HIV-exposed children), including children in whom an HIV diagnosis has been confirmed (OGAC, 2006c). Although prioritization and selection of the activities in the preventive care package for children (0–14 years old) is country-specific, PEPFAR recommends the following components: diagnosis of HIV infection in infants and young children, childhood immunizations, prevention of serious infections, and provision of nutritional care. PEPFAR's activities include efforts to increase early identification of HIV exposure and infection status in children. In the FY2009 annual report to Congress, PEPFAR indicated its support in "expanding polymerase chain reaction (PCR) testing to identify the presence of HIV" including "country-level policy change to allow PCR-based dried blood spot testing," which is thought to reduce the cost and burden of infant diagnosis (OGAC, 2009a, p. 49).

PEPFAR also supports clinical pediatric care for children through various sites—facilities and community- or home-based settings—including the prevention and treatment of OIs, TB, and other diseases like malaria and diarrhea through the provision of pharmaceuticals, ITNs, safe water interventions, and related laboratory services (OGAC, 2009a, 2009e). Moreover, PEPFAR supports palliative care interventions for children and adolescents, including pain and symptom relief using age-appropriate interventions and methods of administration for pediatric palliative care (ages 0–14) (OGAC, 2006d). This includes psychological, social, and spiritual support services intended to alleviate the burden of families caring for family members living with HIV/AIDS, particularly for children and adolescents who often are forced to drop out of school to become the breadwinners of the household and care for the ill parent (OGAC, 2009a). Other critical factors in the care of children are nutrition and growth; therefore, the PEPFAR-supported preventative pediatric care package recommends services that address nutritional needs, such as therapeutic or supplementary feeding, replacement feeding, and provision of micronutrient supplements (OGAC, 2006c). Through the new Five-Year Strategy, PEPFAR II emphasizes the need for governments "to expand coverage, and access to quality basic care packages" for people diagnosed with HIV, including HIV-infected children and adolescents, "particularly through integration of care with other health and development programming" (OGAC, 2009i, p. 18). This is especially significant within the current efforts to guarantee the health and survival of children through referrals and follow-up of HIV-infected children for immunizations, as in the case of many PEPFAR-supported care and PMTCT programs linking services to maternal-child health programs (OGAC, 2009c).

*Programs for Orphans and Vulnerable Children*

In its guidance document, PEPFAR defines orphans and vulnerable children as children who are "either orphaned or made more vulnerable because of HIV/AIDS." Further, it defines an orphan as a child who "has lost one or both parents to HIV/AIDS" (OGAC, 2006e, p. 2). A vulnerable child is defined as a child being "more vulnerable because of any or all of the following factors that result from HIV/AIDS: is HIV-positive; lives without adequate adult support (e.g., in a household with chronically ill parents, a household that has experienced a recent death from chronic illness, a household headed by a grandparent, and/or a household headed by a child); lives outside of family care (e.g., in residential care or on the streets); or is marginalized, stigmatized, or discriminated against" (OGAC, 2006e, p. 2). Because children and adolescents can differ greatly in their needs and individual vulnerabilities, in the past 6 years, PEPFAR has supported "child-centered, family-focused, community-based, and government-supported" OVC programming for these groups in need of further care to facilitate age-appropriate development (OGAC, 2006e, 2009i, p. 22). Therefore, PEPFAR's OVC programs target different age groups of orphans and vulnerable children and adolescents from age 0 to 17 years (see Table 4).

**TABLE 4** PEPFAR Age Categories for Programs for Orphans and Vulnerable Children

| Age | Stage |
| --- | --- |
| <2 years | Infancy |
| 2–4 | Early Childhood/Toddler |
| 5–11 | Middle Childhood |
| 12–17 | Late Childhood/Adolescence |

SOURCE: OGAC (2006e).

In addition to these age groups, the expanded program goals under the new Five-Year Strategy highlight the importance of refocusing OVC program efforts to also address the needs of several neglected subset populations such as young adults, and in particular the vulnerability of girls (see the Gender section of this report) (OGAC, 2009g). According to this strategic plan, PEPFAR will help countries to develop initiatives that target "adolescent and young adults as they transition from OVC programs into society and careers" (OGAC, 2009i, p. 23).

PEPFAR guidance provides an operational definition and guiding principles for OVC programming decisions; nonetheless "each community will need to prioritize those children most vulnerable and in need of further care" (OGAC, 2006e, p. 2). PEPFAR countries use the Child Status Index tool (MEASURE Evaluation, 2009), developed by Duke University and MEASURE Evaluation with USG support, to assist in-country planning of OVC programming based on these core elements and 12 measurable factors that approximate a standard for child health and well-being (OGAC, 2009a).

PEPFAR's OVC programming guidance identifies important elements of a child's and adolescent's life in seven core areas that are based on the principles of the "Framework for the Protection, Care, and Support of Orphans and Vulnerable Children Living in a World with HIV and AIDS" (OGAC, 2006e). These factors, described in more detail below, include food and nutritional support, shelter and care, protection, health care, psychosocial support, education and vocational training, and economic opportunity and/or strengthening. PEPFAR also supports OVC programs "that link OVC services with HIV-affected families [through] linkages with PMTCT, palliative care, treatment" (OGAC, 2009e, p. 137). Further, PEPFAR-supported activities under OVC programs include services that directly support orphans and vulnerable children and adolescents as well as their caregivers, families, and community members (OGAC, 2009e). In addition to activities at the level of patient care and the level of the caregiver, PEPFAR also supports activities at the systems level. As emphasized in the new strategic plan, system-wide OVC program activities are aimed at building local, regional, and national capacity to enhance the structures and networks that support healthy child development. This includes efforts by PEPFAR to assist countries in coordinating among ministries overseeing education, social welfare, and health in order to develop policy and program responses that lead to comprehensive and effective care for orphans and vulnerable children and adolescents (OGAC, 2009i).

**Food and nutritional support** OVC programs include nutritional assessments and counseling, therapeutic or supplementary feeding and micronutrient supplementation for HIV-infected children based on national and appropriate international guidelines, and replacement feeding and support for children born to HIV-infected mothers (OGAC, 2006e). Orphans and vulnerable children are one of the priority groups identified by PEPFAR to receive food and nutritional support. In FY2008, PEPFAR reported that 814,800 orphans and vulnerable children received support for food and nutritional supplementation in the 15 focus countries (OGAC, 2009a). PEPFAR-supported efforts to provide food and nutritional support use linkages with non-HIV funding mechanisms, such as USAID Title II (Food for Peace program[41]) and the United Nations World Food Program as well as programs in partner countries (OGAC, 2006g). In FY2010 PEPFAR's COP Guidance introduced new budget codes for food and nutrition commodities, policy, tools, and service delivery in order to capture information on country activities under this cross-cutting issue (OGAC, 2009a, 2009e). Currently, the only indicator for OVC programs required by OGAC captures the number of eligible individuals under 18 years old who received food and nutrition services (OGAC, 2009d).

**Shelter and care** Because of the growing number of orphans and vulnerable children and adolescents globally, it is necessary to enhance the capacity of families and communities to care for these children. PEPFAR funds can support shelter and care interventions such as: identifying potential caregivers prior to a guardian's death, family tracing and fostering, providing access to temporary shelter for children in transition, supporting child- or adolescent-headed households in taking care of their homes, supporting access to programs that incentivize adoption or the provision of foster care, and strengthening community-based and family-based care models for children (OGAC, 2006e).

**Protection** PEPFAR OVC programs addressing this core area may focus on interventions such as: health care and social services facilitating basic birth registration and identification, the provision of community-based assistance to orphans and vulnerable children for inheritance claims, the removal of children from abusive situations into safe temporary or permanent placements, and the strengthening of local community structures that are responsible for monitoring and protecting orphans and vulnerable children (OGAC, 2006e).

**Health care** Core services for orphans and vulnerable children address (1) the general health needs of this group, (2) health care for HIV-positive children, and (3) prevention of HIV. OVC programs are required to disaggregate health requirements and interventions by age, and they

---

[41] The Food for Peace program (Public Law 480, also renamed Food for Peace Act of 2008) is the principal mechanism through which the USG implements its international food assistance. Title II of the Food for Peace Act, which authorizes the vast majority of U.S. international food assistance, is managed by the USAID Office of Food for Peace. USAID Peace's implementing partners include private voluntary organizations registered with USAID, local and international nongovernmental organizations, and the United Nations World Food Program (USAID, 2009a).

should facilitate access to primary health care for orphans and vulnerable children (OGAC, 2006e). "General health" interventions include: referrals to child health care, the provision of support for survivors of abuse, the training of caregivers to monitor children's health, and capacity building of public and private health providers (OGAC, 2006e). PEPFAR programs provide health care to HIV-positive children, including HIV-exposed children, through direct access to health providers, or through referrals to prevention and treatment services.

**Psychosocial support** Children and adolescents affected by HIV/AIDS suffer anxiety, fear, grief, and trauma with the illness or death of a parent. PEPFAR programs are intended to address the psychosocial and life skills needs of orphans and vulnerable children, including gender-sensitive life skills and experiential learning opportunities; improved links between children affected by HIV/AIDS and their communities; rehabilitation for children who are living outside of family care; and referral to counseling where available and appropriate, particularly for HIV-positive youth (OGAC, 2006e).

**Education and vocational training** Partnerships with the education sector on national and local levels provide an important opportunity to ensure that children and adolescents affected by HIV/AIDS have access to education. Linkages with other programs, such as the USG basic education program or the African Education Initiative (AEI) implemented through USAID, can help expand educational opportunities. For children and adolescents, the USG is providing $400 million through AEI to train 500,000 teachers and provide scholarships for 300,000 children and adolescents, particularly young girls (OGAC, 2009a). Other activities within this core area that are supported by PEPFAR funding include activities that encourage access for orphans and vulnerable children into early childhood development programs, vocational training, activities to integrate orphaned and vulnerable children into community social life, and anti-stigma education. PEPFAR's efforts in this core area also extend to interagency activities, such as the Interagency Education Steering Committee and other strategic planning for the expansion of education wraparound programs that target HIV-infected children and adolescents, as well as those made vulnerable by HIV/AIDS (OGAC, 2009a).

**Economic opportunity and strengthening** PEPFAR programs fund economic strengthening services so that caregivers can meet their responsibilities to ill family members or receive orphaned children into the household. For instance, PEPFAR supports activities that promote the entrepreneurism of caregivers of orphans and vulnerable children through microfinance programs, small-business development, and programs for community-based asset building (OGAC, 2008a). Programs also provide orphans and vulnerable children and adolescents with training and other skills to improve their future economic opportunities (OGAC, 2006e).

## Objective and Scope

The IOM evaluation will assess PEPFAR's progress toward meeting its programmatic targets and strategic goals for children and adolescents, including efforts to increase the number of HIV-infected children receiving treatment and the number of orphans and vulnerable children and adolescents receiving care and support services. Since PEPFAR provides services for children and adolescents through prevention, treatment, and care strategies for children and adolescents, as well as through specific OVC programming, activities in all of these areas, to the extent that they serve children and adolescents, will be a part of the assessment of PEPFAR's effects on the well-being of children and adolescents. The evaluation committee, in its review of PEPFAR-supported programs aimed at the age-specific needs of children and adolescents infected and affected by HIV/AIDS, will consider the appropriateness of programmatic guidance and activities in providing effective care and support to improve the health and psychosocial well-being of these populations. This includes assessing the effect of services provided to children and adolescents in each of the programmatic areas, as well as efforts in supporting family-centered programs and community-led initiatives that respond to the needs of orphans and other vulnerable children and adolescents in PEPFAR countries.

The evaluation committee will consider how PEPFAR's efforts to guide countries to implement international standards of care for children and adolescents, including those orphaned or made vulnerable by HIV/AIDS, have resulted in measurable effects on the well-being of children and adolescents in PEPFAR countries. This will include a review of PEPFAR-supported initiatives such as the development and implementation of national plans for orphans and vulnerable children and other policies related to improving survival and healthy development of children and adolescents.

**Program Impact Pathway**

An impact pathway (Figure 14) summarizes how the IOM evaluation committee proposes to examine the strength of evidence establishing plausible causal links between PEPFAR programs for children and adolescents and their intended impacts. This impact pathway reflects that significant impacts of PEPFAR services in one setting (such as health) may emerge in other service settings (such as education or child welfare). The impact pathway framework will help the committee understand the changes at each stage, in order to describe the relationship between the processes of interventions and their effects. Given the timely availability of data, the evaluation committee will examine whether PEPFAR-funded activities have had an effect on the well-being of children and adolescents through an assessment of mediating output and outcome indicators or intermediate measures of child and adolescent well-being as defined by the committee.

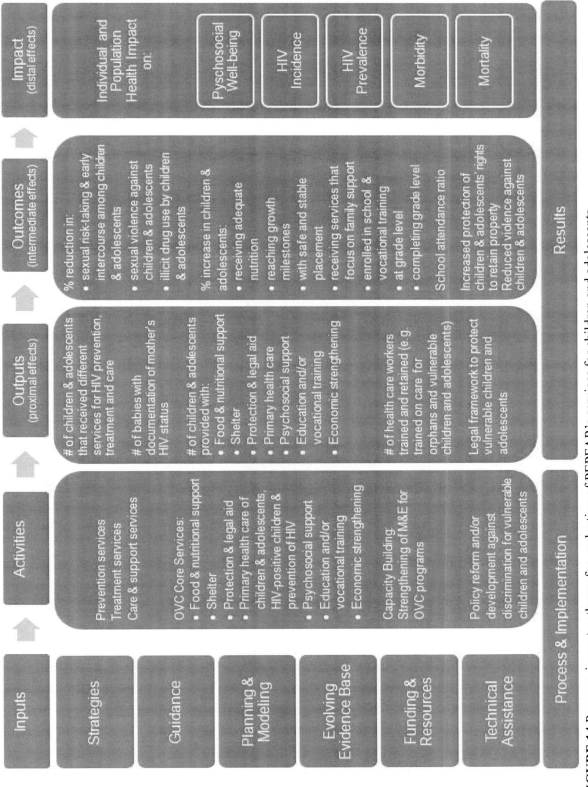

**FIGURE 14** Program impact pathway for evaluation of PEPFAR's services for children and adolescents.

## Illustrative Questions

The limitations in evaluating the effects of PEPFAR's activities on the well-being of children and adolescents include differences in definitions with respect to the age categories of children, adolescent, youth, and young people (UNAIDS Reference Group on Estimates Modelling and Projections, 2002). While PEPFAR defines age-specific categories in some areas, such as pediatric treatment and OVC programming (Table 4), PEPFAR, country-level, and international data-collecting systems do not all use consistent age categories. However, international efforts to harmonize indicators for M&E of interventions targeting these populations, including orphans and vulnerable children under the age of 18 years, will provide some data for the evaluation of PEPFAR activities.

Another potential limitation is the limited availability of age-disaggregated data for many key outcome indicators. The evaluation committee will review program-level data and country-level data to seek sources of age-disaggregated data. However, although countries are increasingly collecting age- and sex-disaggregated data systematically from programs, in particular from those strategically targeting children and adolescents, in many places there still are not enough data to assess and evaluate these programs (UNICEF, 2009). This will be an important issue not only for this evaluation but also during the implementation of PEPFAR II, in particular within the context of implementation plans for partnership frameworks, which under the reauthorization legislation need to contain age- and sex- disaggregated data for "an identification of the intended beneficiaries [...] including information on orphans and vulnerable children, to the maximum extent practicable."[42] In their latest review of PEPFAR-supported care and support activities for children and adolescents, PEPFAR's Pediatric TWG indicated that data on current progress in care and support are not disaggregated by age, HIV exposure, or infection status (OGAC, 2009c). Moreover, they indicate that international indicators, such as UNAIDS globally harmonized indicators, provide only data on scale-up and coverage of particular priority program elements and limited data on receipt of care and support services by HIV-infected children (OGAC, 2009c).

Finally, OVC programs may be offered within different settings in which eligible children and adolescents may receive multiple services. This means that there is a risk of a single child being counted several times by different implementing partners, which can make it difficult to determine if targets expressed as "number of children receiving services" are being met (OGAC, 2009d). The lack of unique identifiers for each participant in PEPFAR activities constitutes a major methodological challenge for program evaluations in this context.

The following are examples of questions that the committee will consider in the evaluation. These questions are intended to contribute to addressing part B, items v, vi, and vii of the areas for consideration in the congressional mandate.[43]

*How are services supported by PEPFAR tailored to the cultural context for the children and adolescents presenting with needs? Specifically, how are these activities tailored or*

---

[42] *Supra.*, note 6 at §301(d)(2), 22 U.S.C. §2151-b2(e)(2)(E)(iv).

[43] (B)(v) an evaluation of the impact of prevention programs on HIV incidence in relevant population groups
(B)(vi) an evaluation of the impact on child health and welfare of interventions authorized under this Act on behalf of orphans and vulnerable children
(B)(vii) an evaluation of the impact of programs and activities authorized in this Act on child mortality

CHILD AND ADOLESCENT WELL-BEING
111

*targeted to specific age cohorts among populations of children and adolescents orphaned and made vulnerable by HIV/AIDS?*

The committee will try to assess the cultural sensitivity and age-appropriateness of PEPFAR programs as they attempt to address culturally entrenched beliefs and practices that increase the risk-taking behavior of children and adolescents orphaned or made vulnerable by HIV/AIDS. The committee will rely on qualitative data to ensure that interventions for children are contextually relevant and that PEPFAR program interventions are responsive to variances in high and low HIV prevalence areas.

*What criteria are used by PEPFAR countries to establish priorities and determine the balance among prevention, treatment, and care interventions for HIV-infected infants, children, and adolescents including those orphaned or made vulnerable by HIV/AIDS?*

*How effective are multi-sector strategic planning and implementation for child and adolescent intervention efforts?*

*Is PEPFAR engaging social, behavioral, and prevention scientists in guiding programs, strategies, and analysis targeting infants, children, and adolescents?*

According to PEPFAR's stated goals, treatment as well as care and support programming targeting HIV-infected children need to be consistent with the pediatric HIV burden in a community but also with the country's continuing sustainability of PEPFAR programs. In order to address these goals, the committee will need to understand how funding priorities are determined for these three main program areas with regard to children and adolescents. The committee will seek to understand the different funding allocation decisions within these programmatic areas, as well as changes in funding over time, through a review of PEPFAR's operational plans and a sample of the COPs. Key informant interviews during country visits will be a complementary source of information.

*What is the responsiveness and adequacy of psychosocial care services to meet the needs of eligible HIV-positive children and adolescents orphaned or made vulnerable by HIV/AIDS?*

PEPFAR recommends countries collect data on the number of orphans and vulnerable children provided with psychological, social, or spiritual support. The committee will rely on qualitative data to assess the "responsiveness and adequacy" of these services as programs do not provide relevant quality data to address these specific issues. To address PEPFAR's efforts in this core OVC program area, the committee will try to evaluate the responsiveness, screening, and referral of children and adolescents to appropriate psychosocial support providers at different stages of need. Efforts will also be made to evaluate the engagement of expert guidance by country programs in determining best practices for addressing the psychosocial needs of children and adolescents orphaned or made vulnerable by HIV/AIDS.

*To what extent have PEPFAR-supported OVC programs had an effect on the educational enrollment of orphans and vulnerable children and adolescents?*

*Are PEPFAR efforts supporting policy or programs aimed at mitigating the consequences of children and adolescents, particularly young women, having increasing socioeconomic responsibilities in the household due to the illness of a parent or both parents living with HIV/AIDS?*

*To what extent are programs averting orphanhood and over what period of time?*

*What economic support programs are in place to generate income for adult non-parental caregivers to support orphans and vulnerable children and adolescents in their households?*

The committee will review available data to assess other cross-cutting socioeconomic interventions such as vocational and technical training, small-business development, and household economic-strengthening workshops. The committee will need to access data disaggregated by age and sex in order to assess the effects of PEPFAR's economic strengthening programs on the socioeconomic needs of these groups at different developmental stages, particularly in young women.

*What activities does PEPFAR support for in-service training and pre-service training for child and adolescent service providers and facilities?*

The long term benefits of PEPFAR on the well-being of children and adolescents, including those orphaned or made vulnerable by HIV, will largely depend on the capacity of country programs to assume responsibility for lessening the negative effects of HIV/AIDS in the communities where they live. Thus, the committee will assess qualitative and quantitative data to evaluate whether PEPFAR programs are investing in building the capacity of district and national authorities and communities to respond to the needs of these vulnerable groups.

*What is the current state of child protection legislation in the community? Are activities supported by PEPFAR contributing to changes in implementation and enforcement?*

Some of the PEPFAR-supported activities include training workshops on children's rights, as well as will writing and succession planning for children, their guardians, and for PEPFAR program staff. PEPFAR programs also link children, adolescents, and their guardians to appropriate legal services. The committee will seek to assess the effects of PEPFAR activities on current or proposed legislative reforms that incorporate child and adolescent protection measures and support protection programs mainly through primary collection of qualitative data during country visits and a review of publicly available documents.

*To what extent have PEPFAR policy initiatives contributed to changes in national health priorities for children and adolescents?*

*Are PEPFAR efforts resulting in the development and adoption of national strategic plans for orphans and vulnerable children? What has been the progress of the country programs to implement the plans?*

A primary measure will be whether PEPFAR programs for children and adolescents orphaned or made vulnerable by HIV/AIDS are an integral part of national HIV/AIDS strategies and plans. The committee will review a range of policy documents (see Box 2a-d) and conduct interviews to assess whether these strategies and/or planning activities are designed to engage different sectors or agencies within the national government dedicated to child and adolescent well-being. The committee will seek any available data from OGAC and governments such as partnership framework implementation plans.

# SECTION 7: GENDER-RELATED VULNERABILITY AND RISK

The global HIV/AIDS epidemic cannot be fully addressed without considering the ways in which societal gender norms, which can be described as "how societies define acceptable and customary roles, responsibilities, and behavior of women, girls, men, and boys," contribute to women's and men's vulnerability in the epidemic (AIDSTAR-One, 2009, p. 1). For example, gender inequalities can limit the ability of women to exert control over their sexual choices, while societal norms may encourage men to engage in riskier sexual behavior. Norms can inhibit access for both men and women to obtain testing and treatment due to, for example, fear of reprisal by a partner or the nature of service provision. In addition, socially defined responsibilities may lead to an increased burden, typically for women, associated with caring for individuals affected by HIV and AIDS (UNIFEM, 2006). A focus on gender inequality and how to reduce it thus has been recognized to be an essential ingredient of HIV prevention, treatment, and care. Current priorities among stakeholders in the global HIV/AIDS community in reducing gender-related vulnerabilities are focused on a variety of country-level strategies. These include the passage and implementation of legislation to protect women, girls, and other vulnerable groups (such as MSM) from gender-based violence, bias, discrimination, and stigma; programs to address male norms; and efforts to empower women through increasing their income generation opportunities (AIDSTAR-One, 2009; UNAIDS, 2010a; UNIFEM, 2006).

This section provides a brief background on gender-related programming in the context of PEPFAR and outlines the committee's approach to assessing PEPFAR's efforts toward addressing these complex issues. However, it is important to note that unlike other aspects of addressing HIV and AIDS, issues associated with gender-related risk and vulnerability cut across all of PEPFAR's implementation, and do not currently comprise their own unique programmatic or funding category. In addition, while ongoing efforts to highlight the differential needs of men and women have been underway since the beginning of the program, addressing issues associated with gender norms, violence, and stigma are still in the early stages in many PEPFAR countries.

## PEPFAR's Efforts on Gender to Date

The original legislation authorizing the creation of PEPFAR and the first Five-Year Strategy acknowledged the importance of addressing the unique vulnerability of women and girls, most notably through prevention efforts, but did not outline any specific targets for addressing gender-related issues (OGAC, 2004). Recognizing the centrality of gender inequality in the AIDS epidemic, PEPFAR subsequently convened a gender TWG in 2005 and submitted a report to Congress on gender-based violence and other gender programming activities in 2006, which emphasized the need to address challenges beyond those associated with access to care, including gender norms and linking services to reduce HIV risk among victims of gender-based violence (OGAC, 2006f).

The Lantos–Hyde Act of 2008 expanded the program's mandate with respect to women and called for the development of a plan to address the particular vulnerability of women and girls and improve research in areas related to gender programming. Working from the reauthorization legislation, the gender TWG also emphasized the following five strategic areas to guide program development and implementation (OGAC, 2009c):

1.  Increasing gender equitable access to prevention activities and services
2.  Reducing violence against women, coercion, and the exploitation of women and girls by sex trafficking, rape and sexual abuse and providing post-rape prophylaxis
3.  Addressing male norms and behaviors
4.  Increasing women's legal rights and protections
5.  Increasing women's access to income and productive resources

The recently released new PEPFAR Five-Year Strategy reaffirmed the program's commitment to gender equity in its prevention, treatment, and care services and to scaling up programs to address gender-based violence (OGAC, 2009g). It also commits the program to work with countries in establishing initial targets and reporting mechanisms to track outcomes for activities targeted at gender needs (OGAC, 2009h).

## Objective and Scope

The IOM evaluation committee will examine the progress made toward incorporating the ideals laid out by the reauthorization legislation and Five-Year Strategy into program guidance, planning, and budgeting processes. The committee will also assess the extent to which PEPFAR has increased its gender programming to include activities aimed at reducing gender-based violence, addressing male norms, empowering women through behavior change and income generating activities, and improving equity in access to prevention, treatment, and care services.

## Program Impact Pathway

The following impact pathway (Figure 15) illustrates the committee's understanding of how activities consistent with PEPFAR's stated overarching gender goals could lead to outputs, outcomes, and health impacts in the countries in which PEPFAR operates. As described in the previous section, efforts to address gender-related issues are still being developed in many countries and are not incorporated in a systematic manner into country program planning. Thus, the activities listed do not represent PEPFAR-wide initiatives, but rather serve as examples of programs that might be undertaken, or are already underway as pilots in some PEPFAR countries. Due to these realities, the committee's assessment will focus primarily on the process of developing gender-related activities and, where possible, the outputs achieved from their implementation. However, the ability to access data on outputs is expected to vary substantially by country and may not be feasible in many settings. The committee may also pursue data from external sources (including from multilateral partners such as UNAIDS), existing studies, and qualitative analysis during country visits.

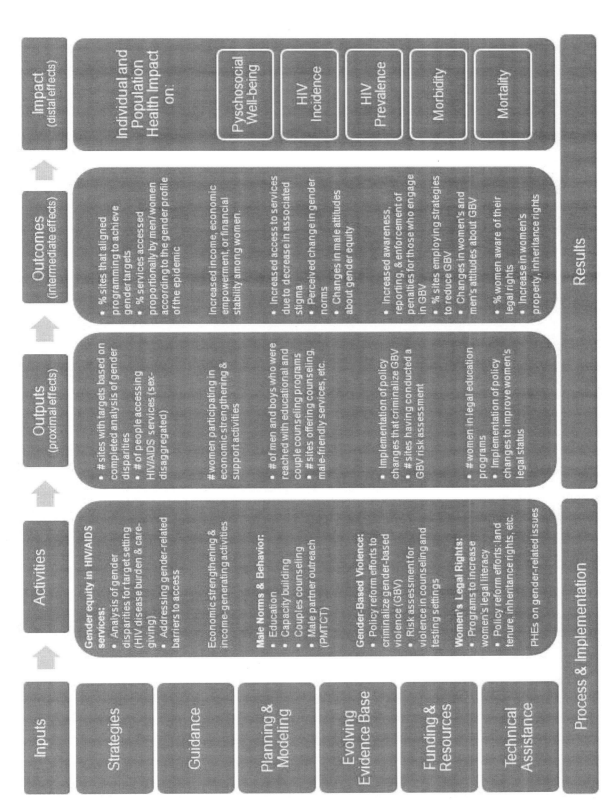

**FIGURE 15** Program impact pathway for evaluation of PEPFAR's gender efforts.
NOTES: PHE = public health evaluations; PMTCT = prevention of mother-to-child transmission.

## Illustrative Questions

The following are illustrative examples of the types of questions related to gender activities that the committee may assess given the timely availability of quality data. These questions are intended to contribute to addressing part B, item vii of the areas for consideration in the congressional mandate.[44]

There are currently no PEPFAR reported, required, or recommended indicators that are specific to measuring efforts toward changes in gender norms, vulnerability related to gender, or empowerment. However, a number of prevention, treatment, and care indicators are required to be disaggregated by sex and/or age, which can provide information related to access rates and equity in service provision. In addition, due to potential variability in the definition and understanding of gender-related activities across programs, there will likely be substantial variation both within and between countries. As this represents an evolving area of programming, case studies may provide useful information at this stage.

*Are women and girls accessing prevention, treatment, and care programs in equal numbers to men and boys?*

Sex-disaggregated PEPFAR indicators (such as the number of people accessing prevention, treatment, and care programs) will be used where available. The committee may also assess whether these services are being delivered in a comparable and appropriate manner to women and men, using qualitative data collected during country visits.

*Has PEPFAR made special efforts to reduce the sexual risk of adolescent girls and young women (e.g., through early marriage, transactional, or cross-generational sex, etc.)? Has PEPFAR made efforts to address the sexual risk of older women (e.g., through wife inheritance by relatives of late brothers, cleansing rites, etc.)? Have these efforts been successful?*

As with assessing male norms, the committee may use structured interviews with key informants from the OGAC, program, and project levels to determine the incorporation of efforts to reduce women's sexual risk into program planning and implementation. When available at the country level, the committee will pursue access to a limited number of recommended PEPFAR indicators, including those related to cross-generational sex. In addition, there are a number of global level indicators collected by organizations and survey efforts (including UNAIDS, national demographic and health surveys, and behavioral surveillance surveys) that provide information regarding this topic (Measure DHS, 2010). The committee will assess the feasibility of incorporating information from these types of sources to provide contextual data on the countries in which PEPFAR operates.

*How many programs integrate or are linked to programs that seek to economically empower women? What has been their impact in improving women's income, savings, or access to credit?*

---

[44] (B)(iii) an assessment of efforts to address gender-specific aspects of HIV/AIDS, including gender related constraints to accessing services and addressing underlying social and economic vulnerabilities of women and men

Currently, activities that promote economic empowerment and income generation are included under the umbrella of care services provided by PEPFAR, and indicators such as "number of people provided with a minimum of one care service" disaggregated by sex may provide some information as to the existence of these programs. However, in order to gain a more comprehensive picture of the success and coverage of these types of activities, the committee will seek other sources of data at the project level where available.

*How many programs has PEPFAR supported to address male norms and behaviors? What criteria are used to determine whether such programs should be a part of a COP? How effective have these programs been in fostering more gender equitable attitudes among men?*

The availability of activity type data at the OGAC level will determine the committee's ability to assess the efforts of PEPFAR toward addressing male norms. Interviews with OGAC, country, and project level staff may be used to determine how these types of activities are addressed in the program planning and reporting process. However, there are no PEPFAR indicators for measuring impact of programs to change male behavior or norms. Thus, the evaluation committee will use project level data where it exists.

*How many country programs include programs to reduce gender-based violence? How and to what extent have they succeeded in reducing incidence of violence?*

There are no PEPFAR indicators specific to measuring gender-based violence, so the committee will use country data and project level data where it is available. Data may also be gathered from key informants who run these programs. In addition, the committee will attempt to follow-up at the OGAC level on the "Report on Gender-Based Violence and HIV/AIDS" that was submitted to Congress in 2006, to assess the potential of updating the information presented.

*Has PEPFAR made efforts to influence national policy and legal environments that affect the vulnerability of women and girls? How have they been successful? What impact have these efforts had on decreasing this vulnerability?*

Efforts toward positively influencing policy and legal reform efforts will be assessed through interviews with country team and OGAC staff. In addition, for the countries for which they have been completed, the newly formed Partnership Frameworks may be reviewed for the presence of gender-related strategies as they are intended to reflect national political and legal priorities. Given the often protracted nature of policy implementation and enforcement, an evaluation of the potential impact of these efforts may not be feasible.

# SECTION 8: KEY SYSTEMS-LEVEL GOALS AND ACTIVITIES

## Reauthorization Legislation Shifts Priority to Sustainability

The Lantos–Hyde Act of 2008 specifically required PEPFAR's strategy to "include a longer-term estimate of the projected resource needs to progress toward greater sustainability and country ownership of HIV/AIDS programs […] during the 10-year period beginning on October 1, 2013."[45] The new PEPFAR Five-Year Strategy stated that management of the response to the disease and its effects must increasingly be led by countries, with support from bilateral and multilateral partners. Countries also need to increasingly own the process of monitoring, evaluating, and responding to the unique characteristics of the epidemic in their country (OGAC, 2009g). This section therefore outlines how the evaluation committee will explore the role of PEPFAR programs in facilitating improvements to health systems in partner countries and the readiness of PEPFAR and partner countries to increasingly share responsibility for managing the response to the epidemic and move to greater sustainability and country ownership.

*Definitions*

Neither the authorizing legislation nor the PEPFAR strategy defines sustainability. For the purposes of this evaluation, one of several definitions proposed by the OECD Development Assistance Committee may be used; it defines sustainability as "the continuation of benefits from a development intervention after major development assistance has been completed" (DAC Network on Development Evaluation, 2002).

While continuation of benefits into the future is the ultimate goal, a number of intermediate outputs or outcomes can be posited to improve sustainability:

- Affordability: The extent to which countries can bear the cost of programs.
- Efficiency/cost-effectiveness: "A measure of how economically resources/inputs (funds, expertise, time, etc.) are converted to results" (DAC Network on Development Evaluation, 2002, p. 21).
- Country capacity: The ability of government, the private sector, and civil society to "plan, manage, implement, and account for results of policies and programs" (High-Level Forum, 2005, p. 5).[46]
- Country "ownership": A situation in which "partner countries exercise effective leadership over their development policies and strategies, and coordinate development actions"(High-Level Forum, 2005, p. 3).
- Coordination and harmonization[47] with donors and governments: The extent to which donors "implement, where feasible, common arrangements at country level for planning, funding (e.g., joint financial arrangements), disbursement, monitoring, evaluating and reporting to government on donor activities and aid flows." (High-Level Forum, 2005, p. 6).

---

[45] *Supra.*, note 6 §101(a), 22 U.S.C. §7611(a)(29).
[46] The Paris Declaration does not specify whose capacity within countries this defines, but it is inferred to be the government's capacity. Thus, this proposed definition is somewhat broader.
[47] As the extent to which PEPFAR has contributed to harmonization is being evaluated by the U.S. Government Accountability Office, it will not be explicitly addressed in this proposed evaluation.

*Partnership Frameworks to Promote Sustainable Approaches*

The Lantos–Hyde Act of 2008 permitted the USG to establish framework documents (Partnership Frameworks) with countries to promote a more sustainable approach of the USG's global efforts against HIV/AIDS, malaria, and TB "that is characterized by strengthened country capacity, ownership, and leadership" (OGAC, 2009b, p. 3). Further, these 5-year joint strategic frameworks between the USG and partner governments are meant to intensify focus on cooperation through "technical assistance and support for service delivery, policy reform, and coordinated financial commitments" (OGAC, 2009b, p. 3). At the end of the 5-year time frame, the expectation is that "country governments will be better positioned to assume primary responsibility for the national response to HIV/AIDS in terms of management, strategic direction, performance monitoring, decision making, coordination, and where possible, financial support and service delivery" (OGAC, 2009b, p. 3). The axiom of "do no harm" has been adopted by OGAC for continued support of existing implementing partner service delivery systems to continue to provide quality services while this transition to county ownership occurs over time. There are additional expectations of transparency, accountability, and engagement of multiple stakeholders in the country.

As for policy reform and financial commitments, the Partnership Frameworks are supposed to emphasize policy areas identified by the government and civil society that require additional or focused attention and overall accountability for resources and appropriate budgeting in HIV programs. They also provide a capacity building opportunity for the USG to assist countries in managing multiple funding sources. Some countries, based on their resources, are expected to increase their financial contributions over time. The Partnership Frameworks also provide an opportunity for the USG to provide technical assistance to countries for improved monitoring and tracking of overall health spending (including HIV/AIDS) from different sources, including financial monitoring and reporting systems (OGAC, 2009b).

Although the reauthorization legislation did not define sustainability *per se*, PEPFAR did define how to promote sustainability in the Partnership Frameworks and Partnership Framework Implementation Plans guidance issued in September 2009—based on the principles of the Three Ones, the Paris Declaration, and the Monterey Accord of 2002 (activities that facilitate financing for development): "For purposes of the Partnership Frameworks, promoting sustainability means supporting the partner government in growing its capacity to lead, manage, and ultimately finance its health system with indigenous resources (including its civil society sector), rather than external resources, to the greatest extent possible" (OGAC, 2009b, p. 4). The Partnership Frameworks are distinct from the annual work plans for USG-supported intervention, the COPs. However, COPs are expected to reflect the Partnership Framework principles and the transition strategy outlined in the Partnership Framework Implementation Plans. The implementation plans have minimal required elements, including "an analysis of how the existing portfolio of USG-supported, NGO-implemented programs will transition to the partner government, remain NGO-based, or be terminated within the 5-year timeframe" (OGAC, 2009b, p. 6) and "a description of the approach to supporting increased country ownership, baseline data, specific strategies for achieving the 5-year goals and objectives, and a monitoring and evaluation plan" (OGAC, 2009b, p. 8). It also seems reasonable that cost efficiencies for the future national response can be identified by both PEPFAR and the partner government during the implementation of the Partnership Frameworks and by the end of the 5-year performance period, when countries are expected to assume primary responsibility for the national HIV/AIDS response, even if the partner government does not assume full responsibility of financing its health system.

The goals and objectives would be measureable goals for the USG and all partners in the Partnership Framework. As such, the Partnership Frameworks are expected to identify indicators to assess progress toward meeting the goals, objectives, and programmatic and financial commitments—with an eye toward international efforts to harmonize indicators. PEPFAR-specific reporting systems are expected to be transitioned to nationally- and country-owned systems. This step would be in full support of the Third One—one agreed HIV/AIDS country-level M&E system (OGAC, 2009b). Lastly, the guidance also states that country governments should be developing the "capacity to support all relevant components … of a multi-sector health system" (OGAC, 2009b, p. 4). These components are the six areas of the WHO six-building block framework for effective health systems (see Figure 16) that has been endorsed by PEPFAR.

## Program and Health System Interaction and Integration

The most widely accepted definition of a health system was proposed by the WHO—"all organizations, people, and actions whose primary intent is to promote, restore, or maintain health" (WHO, 2007a, p. 2). A health system therefore includes both public and private (for-profit and not-for-profit) providers, which may be either community- or facility-based. Identifying both well-planned synergies and unintended antagonisms with national health systems that may have resulted from the implementation of a program like PEPFAR requires a systems model, as interventions in one part of the health system may have impacts in others. The WHO Positive Synergies working group took such an approach, resulting in several recommendations that are relevant to PEPFAR: prioritize health system strengthening, agree on and track health system strengthening indicators, align resource allocation between global health initiatives and country health systems, generate more reliable data for the costs and benefits of strengthening health systems, and commit to increased national and global health financing that is more predictable to support sustainable and equitable growth of health systems (Samb et al., 2009).

While global HIV prevalence stabilized in 2000 (Bongaarts et al., 2008; UNAIDS, 2008), the absolute burden of HIV treatment demand will continue to grow each year for the foreseeable future. (UNAIDS, 2008; UNAIDS and WHO, 2009). With newly-infected people still outpacing both AIDS-related deaths and numbers of people being put on ART, it is increasingly clear that treatment alone will not be a sufficient response to control the epidemic (Bertozzi et al., 2009). Achieving sustainable HIV programs not only requires health system strengthening, but also successful scale-up of effective HIV prevention strategies to avert continued growth in the HIV treatment burden in health systems that are already overburdened. As previously mentioned in the Mapping of PEPFAR Funding section, scaling-up does not necessarily mean just increased spending, so understanding unit costs of HIV-program delivery may help elucidate variation in health system capacity, efficiencies, and quality. Also program and data management and health information systems are needed to more completely assess population impact rather than just process measures.

## Capacity Building

As has been noted, the capacity to scale up programs in low-income countries is limited by resource constraints, including lack of trained health workers and fragile health systems. PEPFAR II therefore added an additional target of training 140,000 new health workers to support the capacity of countries to improve "the overall quality of their services … and build capacity to plan, manage and sustainably finance their health systems" (OGAC, 2009h). Investing in healthcare workers and health systems increases the likelihood of more people receiving prevention and treatment services for HIV and of achieving a broader health impact (PEPFAR Reauthorization Action Team, 2010).

## Joint Activities Between PEPFAR and the Global Fund

As seen in the statement of task in Appendix A, Congress mandates the committee to evaluate the impact on health of prevention, treatment, and care efforts that are supported by U.S. funding, including multilateral and bilateral programs involving joint operations. Further discussions among IOM staff, OGAC, and congressional staff[48] clarified "multilateral and bilateral programs involving joint operations" to mean programs operated in conjunction with bilateral funding through PEPFAR and the Global Fund (Bressler, 2009; Marsh, 2009). In the preliminary research of the planning committee, this includes financing of ART and procurement and supply management of ARVs and other commodities for its Voluntary Pooled Procurement (discussed in the Adult and Pediatric Treatment section of this report), as well as prevention and care activities (PMTCT and TB treatment, respectively discussed in the Prevention and Care and Support Services sections). It also includes time-limited, outcome-oriented technical assistance through centrally-funded grants from OGAC to Global Fund recipients with active grants (which are not necessarily PEPFAR recipients). The USG Global Fund Technical Support Advisory Panel advises OGAC headquarters on these technical assistance activities.

Begun in 2005 under the Grants Management Solutions project, this technical support is intended to (1) improve the functioning of Global Fund grants, (2) strengthen local capacity, and (3) alleviate specific bottlenecks to address under-performing Global Fund grants. The main areas identified with inadequate or poor performance were organizational development (including governance and leadership), financial management, procurement and supply management, and M&E (Coleman, 2007; PEPFAR, 2009b). These four areas correspond to four of the six blocks in the WHO building-block model for effective health systems (see Figure 16). There are stated goals for improvement for each of the four areas of technical assistance. In July 2008, a USG Global Fund Technical Support Evaluation was conducted, which showed achievements through 2008 in each of the areas from the $12 million available in FY2005 technical support through the $31 million available in FY2007 (Coleman, 2010). The committee will examine the 2008 evaluation, including its methods and findings and will also request available country/recipient progress reports as well as copies of the grant requests from recipient countries.

---

[48] *Supra.*, note 10.

## Evaluation Strategy

As part of an evaluation of the impact of PEPFAR, it is necessary to determine partner country readiness to make this transition to sustainability. To assess partner country readiness, the evaluation committee aims to examine the partnership frameworks with partner countries. In addition, the committee will assess PEPFAR efforts and synergy with other global stakeholders for capacity building and technical assistance, including activities similar to those identified by the International Health Partnership, such as donor funding harmonization and collaboration between international actors and developing countries to develop and implement national health plans.

The committee will also establish working definitions, define data sources, and identify evaluation methodologies for the key parameters of sustainability that include country ownership and local capacity building, including health system strengthening and healthcare workforce expansion. However, it has been noted that "little [global] consensus has emerged to provide uniform guidance" to indicators that can track these activities, although the development of these indicators is an area of intense international interest and activity. PEPFAR defines indicator and reporting requirements in health systems strengthening "to reflect a more narrow scope of interest tied to PEPFAR's focus on HIV" (OGAC, 2009d, p. 199)—resulting in selection of two indicators to be reported centrally to OGAC that reflect laboratory and health workforce strengthening. Evaluating data for other parameters will require metrics not currently available from routine data sources or the PEPFAR indicator database (OGAC, 2009d), including extra-health sector factors such as good governance (Dybul, 2009), to permit the committee to assess performance of current or past PEPFAR activities. The committee will also examine Partnership Frameworks and Implementation Plans to assess what the countries and OGAC are responsible for, how it is being measured or tracked, and how the processes evolve for PEPFAR-related responsibilities and activities to be transitioned to country leadership for sustainable programs and positive impacts on individual and population health.

### Health System Frameworks

PEPFAR's increased focus on health systems is shared with other global health initiatives, including The Global Alliance for Vaccines and Immunisation (2010) and the Global Fund, as well as the World Bank and the WHO. The committee will benefit from and incorporate deliberations among these agencies that will address both how to define health systems and how to measure progress toward strengthened health systems (Frenk, 2010; Shakarishvili, 2009).

Adopting a common conceptual framework is a key requirement for the evaluation of health systems strengthening and is important to framing such measures. The most widely adopted framework, proposed by the WHO in 2007, is based on operational "building blocks" of the health system (Figure 16)—services, workforce, information, commodities and technologies, financing, and leadership/governance (WHO, 2007a). These building blocks serve several functions including describing what a health system should have the capacity to do in each of these blocks to lead to improved health, system responsiveness, improved efficiency, and social and financial risk protection. It also lends itself well to a descriptive set of activities that may be undertaken through PEPFAR programs. The importance of "systems thinking" has also been emphasized, because health systems are complex, dynamic, and non-linear systems whose function is dependent on the interplay of all of its components, including "the spaces in between" (Atun and Menabde, 2008; de Savigny and Taghreed, 2009).

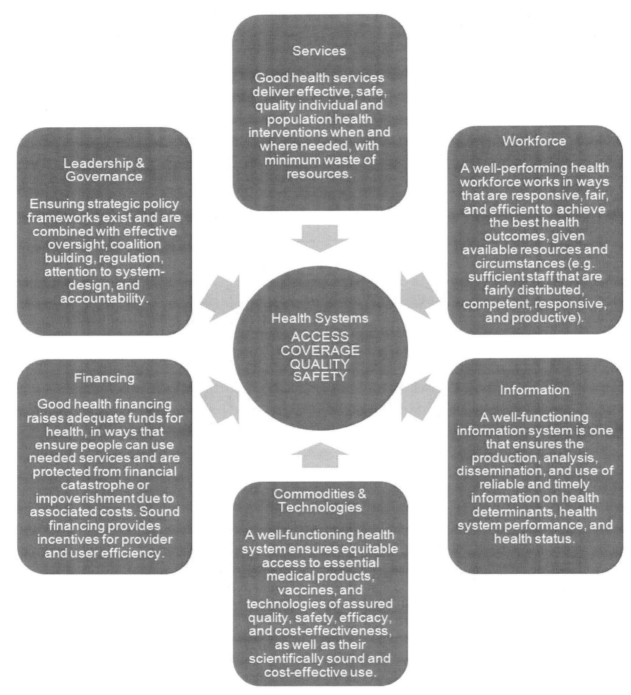

**FIGURE 16** Representation of WHO's six building blocks for effective health systems.
SOURCE: Adapted from WHO, 2007a.

## Program Impact Pathway

The committee will utilize an impact pathway (Figure 17) to assess PEPFAR inputs, output, and outcomes where measurable, within the context of the WHO building blocks framework for health systems strengthening. The pathway can also help assess the same block elements for technical assistance and other activities related to country readiness for assuming increased to total responsibility for their HIV/AIDS response. Although a useful evaluation tool, the linear nature of an impact pathway is a simplified representation of the reality of PEPFAR programs and their impact, and the committee found this to be particularly challenging in the area of systems-level activities. Activities at the systems level are intended to result in an outcome or impact on the health system, but these are also critical inputs to all other programmatic areas. Thus, the functioning of the health system can be both a starting and end point for a pathway. The committee grappled with illustrating the complexities, dynamism, and non-linear nature of health systems with this linear pathway—analogous to forcing a "square peg in a round hole" —but ultimately recognized the utility of the impact pathway to evaluate the process by helping to frame the areas of inquiry and the measures that may be undertaken to assess health system strength. The findings will be interpreted in light of the more complex realities when the evaluation committee draws conclusions and makes recommendations.

As previously mentioned, PEPFAR II (as well as the GHI) has adopted the WHO six building block framework to assess its capacity building and programmatic impact on health systems, categorizing contribution to (1) core HIV activities, (2) secondary benefits or intentional spillover effects of PEPFAR activities on other programs, and (3) targeted leveraging including partnerships.

The six building block elements are denoted in the figure with blocks in all uppercase letters. The committee's working definition of an intervention that strengthens health systems is one that improves the activities and processes within the six health system building blocks, and manages interactions within the "building blocks" over time to achieve more equitable and sustained improvements in population health outcomes. These effects may be either short-term (e.g., better trained workforce delivering higher quality care) or longer-term (e.g., higher-quality care results in a healthier population that is economically more productive), thus growing resources that feed back into the causal chain as an input to the health system. Additional outcomes of an effective health system (e.g., social and financial risk protection for beneficiaries accessing and utilizing services or increased block or system efficiency) can result in increased responsiveness and potentially expanded service coverage when the activities within and among the blocks dynamically interact (see Figure 17). As previously mentioned, interventions in one part of the health system may have impacts in others. Since any intervention may affect the entire system, evaluation is, by definition, context-specific and requires a mix of evaluation strategies, both quantitative and qualitative. Although improved health is an important impact of health systems strengthening, additional measures regarding health system efficiency and equitable distribution of benefits may likewise be important to track as they are developed and adopted by international working groups.

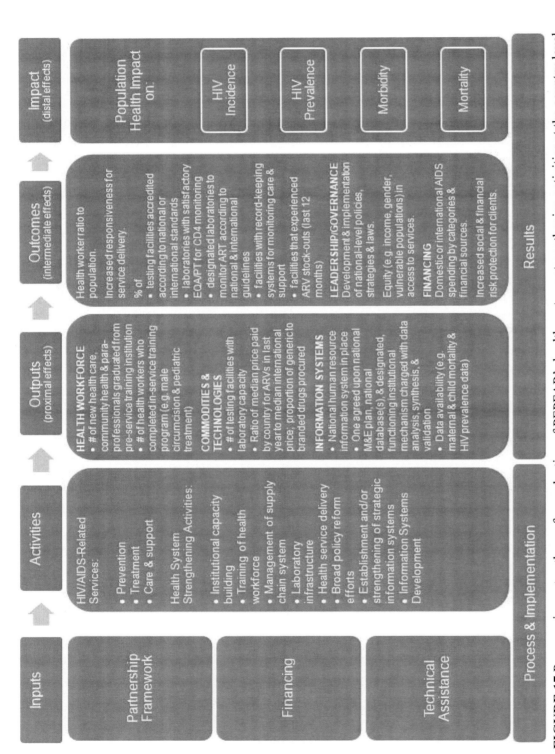

**FIGURE 17** Program impact pathway for evaluation of PEPFAR's health systems strengthening activities at the country level.
NOTES: Upper case headers indicate the WHO's six building blocks. All of the elements listed in the pathway can be categorized under one of the six building blocks, but due to space limitations, select elements were chosen to illustrate blocks within the pathway. ARV = antiretroviral drugs; ART = antiretroviral therapy; CD4 = cluster of differentiation 4; EQA/PT = external quality assurance/proficiency testing; M&E = monitoring and evaluation.

**Illustrative Questions**

The main questions that the committee will consider in the evaluation include the potential positive and negative impact of PEPFAR activities on country-level health system functioning, with regards to both HIV and non-HIV programs. Examples of the kinds of questions the committee may ask that specifically link the WHO six building blocks to our results chain framework include the following. These questions are intended to contribute to addressing part B, item ii of the areas for consideration in the congressional mandate.[49] Because health systems are a fundamental aspect of all program activities, these questions are also intended to contribute to addressing all of the areas for consideration described in the Statement of Task (see Appendix A).

*Finance: To what extent has PEPFAR funding and technical assistance for sound public finance systems resulted in more efficient and equitable care in HIV and non-HIV health systems? To what extent do the joint funds from the Global Fund support the six building blocks? To what extent have the technical support funds from PEPFAR to the Global Fund improved the performance of grant recipients in general and how is this measured? For the four main areas of technical assistance which are among the six WHO building blocks and how are they measured?*

*Commodities and Procurement: How have PEPFAR technical assistance and training affected HIV laboratory diagnostic capacity, pharmacy infrastructure, and supply chain management for reagents and drugs?*

*Information Systems: What is the evidence that PEPFAR-supported health information systems are resulting in higher functioning, quality-driven health systems performance? How will new and existing information officers be trained to meet country needs to strengthen higher functioning and increased quality?*

*Service Delivery: What elements of more efficient, equitable, and effective service delivery should be expected to result in improved population health over time with better integration of HIV- and non-HIV health care and use of continuous quality improvement methods?*

*Leadership and Governance: To what extent will partnership frameworks, jointly funded Global Fund activities, and other expressions of country ownership lead to improved and accountable governance as well as transfer of oversight, management, guidance, and financing for HIV-related services in health systems?*

*Health Workforce: How will the pre-service education target of 140,000 new workers affect health system equity of access (e.g., rural versus urban) and health system strengthening such as increased skill capacity and retention of workforce? Are there other types of workers, (e.g., social service workers and program managers) who also need to be trained? What proportion of newly trained new health or social workers is*

---

[49] (B)(ii) an assessment of the effects on health systems, including on the financing and management of health systems and the quality of service delivery and staffing

*retained one year later? How does PEPFAR support the country's existing health resources development plan or help develop those where absent?*

The committee will also assess progress toward the goals of increased country ownership to transition the HIV/AIDS response to national governments for long-term sustainability. Although there are high-volume discussions within the global development assistance community in this area, there appear to be few to no meaningful metrics to measure increased ownership or country readiness, no accepted logic models to describe and illustrate the transition process, and no indicators for when a country has sufficiently strengthened governance/ leadership or built and operated a financially-sound public finance system to implement and oversee a national health plan. Illustrative questions for this area of the evaluation include the following. Country ownership and sustainability cut across all PEPFAR activities and as such these questions are intended to contribute to addressing all of the areas for consideration in the congressional mandate, as described in the Statement of Task (see Appendix A).

> *How is country ownership defined by the country? By PEPFAR? By relevant global stakeholders in aid development? Are there differences? Have they been reconciled? Do the Partnership Frameworks represent an "agreement" on the definition between the country and PEPFAR?*

> *To what extent have PEPFAR capacity-building, technical assistance, and financing activities to countries contributed to country readiness for transitioning the knowledge management, decision making responsibility, financing, and accountability/oversight of the PEPFAR-funded HIV/AIDS response to the national government? How is it being measured? Are plans in place for future activities needed to improve or increase country readiness if PEPFAR were absent?*

> *How will achievements or milestones by country and/or PEPFAR be measured in the Partnership Frameworks? Will these measures adequately reflect country readiness for program, policy, and financial transitions?*

> *Is the country transitional process explained adequately? Will it be standard for all countries or adapted for each country? Will the transition be parceled over time? Which pieces might be transitioned over time, how, and why?*

> *What are the achievements and lessons learned from the Technical Support Grants to the Global Fund from PEPFAR? How are they measuring whether bottlenecks have been opened or bypassed? What has been the impact on the functioning of programs?*

> *How do Global Fund and PEPFAR measure their relative and unique contributions to programs they jointly fund or operate? How are access, equity, and quality measured for these programs?*

A more extensive listing of illustrative questions for this complex issue that the committee may attempt to address, given the timely availability of quality data, can be found in Appendix H. These may help guide assessment of whether and how PEPFAR has helped countries to mount a stronger response to their HIV epidemics, plan for transition to country ownership including effective leadership and oversight of multilateral donor activities, and focus on affordable care that meets population health needs.

Sustainability and its associated elements must be considered for all of PEPFAR's support. PEPFAR activities will be evaluated relative to their contribution of inputs and support of processes, and the resulting outputs and outcomes. These should ultimately result in the desired outcome of stronger health systems that can more adequately respond not only to HIV but to other serious causes of morbidity and mortality, as well as any emerging challenges to the health and safety of their respective populations.

# REFERENCES

AIDSTAR-One. 2009. *Integrating multiple gender strategies to improve HIV and AIDS interventions: A compendium of programs in Africa.* Washington, DC: International Center for Research on Women.

Alagiri, P., C. Collins, T. Summers, S. Morin, and T. Coates. 2001. *Global spending on HIV/AIDS: Tracking public and private investments in AIDS prevention, care, and research.* Washington, DC: Kaiser Family Foundation.

Atun, R., and N. Menabde. 2008. Health systems and systems thinking. In *Health systems and the challenge of communicable disease,* edited by R. Coker, R. Atun and M. McKee. Berkshire, United Kingdom: Open University Press.

Auvert, B., D. Taljaard, E. Lagarde, J. Sobngwi-Tambekou, R. Sitta, and A. Puren. 2005. Randomized, controlled intervention trial of male circumcision for reduction of HIV infection risk: The ANRS 1265 trial. *PLoS Med* 2(11):e298.

Bailey, R. C., S. Moses, C. B. Parker, K. Agot, I. Maclean, J. N. Krieger, C. F. Williams, R. T. Campbell, and J. O. Ndinya-Achola. 2007. Male circumcision for HIV prevention in young men in Kisumu, Kenya: A randomised controlled trial. *Lancet* 369(9562):643–656.

Bendavid, E., and J. Bhattacharya. 2009. The President's Emergency Plan for AIDS Relief in Africa: An evaluation of outcomes. *Ann Int Med* 150:688–695.

Bertozzi, S. M. 2006. Modeling the impact of antiretroviral use in developing countries. *PLoS Med* 3(4):e148.

Bertozzi, S., T. E. Martz, and P. Piot. 2009. The evolving HIV/AIDS response and the urgent tasks ahead *Health Aff* 28(6):1585.

Bongaarts, J., T. Buettner, G. Heilig, and F. Pelletier. 2008. Has the HIV epidemic peaked? *Popul Dev Rev* 34(2):199–224.

Bouey, P. 2010. *PEPFAR next generation strategic information.* Presentation, Public information-gathering session of the Committee on Planning the Assessment/Evaluation of HIV/AIDS Programs Implemented Under the U.S. Global Leadership Against HIV/AIDS, Tuberculosis, and Malaria Reauthorization Act of 2008, Washington, DC, January 7.

Bressler, S. 2009. Presentation, First Committee Meeting on Planning the Assessment/Evaluation of HIV/AIDS Programs Implemented Under the U.S. Global Leadership Against HIV/AIDS, Tuberculosis, and Malaria Reauthorization Act of 2008, Washington, DC, November 23.

Bush, G. W. 2003. *2003 State of the Union address.* http://georgewbush-whitehouse.archives.gov/news/releases/2003/01/20030128-19.html (accessed June 8, 2010).

Bussmann, H., C. W. Wester, N. Ndwapi, N. Grundmann, T. Gaolathe, J. Puvimanasinghe, A. Avalos, M. Mine, K. Seipone, M. Essex, V. Degruttola, and R. G. Marlink. 2008. Five-year outcomes of initial patients treated in Botswana's national antiretroviral treatment program. *AIDS* 22(17):2303–2311.

CDC (U.S. Centers for Disease Control and Prevention). 1981. Pneumocystis pneumonia—Los Angeles. *MMWR* 30(21):1–3.

CIDA (Canadian International Development Agency). *Project browser.* http://les.acdi-cida.gc.ca/project-browser (accessed June 23, 2010).

Cluver, L., and F. Gardner. 2007. The mental health of children orphaned by AIDS: A review of international and Southern African research. *Child Adolesc Ment Health* 19(1):1–17.

Cluver, L., and M. Orkin. 2009. Stigma, bullying, poverty and AIDS-orphanhood: Interactions mediating psychological problems for children in South Africa. *Soc Sci Med.* 69(8):1186–1193.

Cluver, L., F. Gardner, and D. Operario. 2007. Psychological distress amongst AIDS-orphaned children in urban South Africa. *J Child Psychol Psychiatry* 48(8):755–763.

Coleman, A. 2007. *The U.S. President's Emergency Plan for AIDS Relief: Global Fund technical support*. Presentation, Global Fund Regional Meeting, Nusa Dua, Indonesia, September 3–5. http://www.theglobalfund.org/documents/regionalmeetings/indonesia2007/Presentation_on_ Global_Fund_Technical_Support.ppt (accessed June 14, 2010).

Constella Group LLC. 2008. *Software*. http://constellafutures.com/fg/cdIAC/software.html (accessed April 7, 2010).

Corbett, E. L., C. J. Watt, N. Walker, D. Maher, B. G. Williams, M. C. Raviglione, and C. Dye. 2003. The growing burden of tuberculosis: Global trends and interactions with the HIV epidemic. *Arch Intern Med* 163(9):1009–1021.

Cornman, D. H., S. M. Kiene, S. Christie, W. A. Fisher, P. A. Shuper, S. Pillay, G. H. Friedland, C. M. Thomas, L. Lodge, and J. D. Fisher. 2008. Clinic-based intervention reduces unprotected sexual behavior among HIV-infected patients in Kwazulu-Natal, South Africa: Results of a pilot study. *J Acquir Immune Defic Syndr* 48(5):553–560.

CRS (Congressional Research Service). 2003. *HIV/AIDS international programs: Appropriations, FY2002–FY2004*, edited by R. Copson. Washington, DC: Library of Congress.

CRS . 2005. *The Global Fund and PEPFAR in U.S. international AIDS policy*, edited by R. W. Copson. Order Code RL33135. Washington, DC: CRS.

CRS. 2007. *PEPFAR: From emergency to sustainability*, edited by T. Salaam-Blyther. Order Code RL34192. Washington, DC: CRS.

CRS. 2008a. *International HIV/AIDS, tuberculosis, and malaria: Key changes to U.S. programs and funding*, edited by K. Moss. Order Code RL34569. Washington, DC: CRS.

CRS. 2008b. *Trends in U.S. global AIDS spending: FY2000-FY2008*, edited by T. Salaam-Blyther. Order Code RL33771. Washington, DC: CRS.

CRS. 2009. *PEPFAR reauthorization: Key policy debates and changes to U.S. international HIV/AIDS, tuberculosis, and malaria programs and funding*, edited by K. Moss. Order Code RL34569. Washington, DC: CRS.

Cunningham, C. K., M. L. Chaix, C. Rekacewicz, P. Britto, C. Rouzioux, R. D. Gelber, A. Dorenbaum, J. F. Delfraissy, B. Bazin, L. Mofenson, and J. L. Sullivan. 2002. Development of resistance mutations in women receiving standard antiretroviral therapy who received intrapartum nevirapine to prevent perinatal human immunodeficiency virus type 1 transmission: A substudy of pediatric AIDS clinical trials group protocol 316. *J Infect Dis* 186(2):181–188.

DAC (Development Assistance Committee) Network on Development Evaluation. 2002. *Glossary of key terms in evaluation and results based management, evaluation and aid effectiveness*. Paris: Organisation for Economic Co-operation and Development.

DART Trial Team. 2009. Routine versus clinically driven laboratory monitoring of HIV antiretroviral therapy in Africa (DART): A randomised non-inferiority trial. *Lancet* 375(9709):123–131.

De Lay, P. 2010. *Implementation strategy roundtable: The future of PEPFAR*. Presentation, 17th Conference on Retroviruses and Opportunistic Infections (CROI), San Francisco, CA, February 16–19.

de Savigny, D., and A. Taghreed. 2009. *Systems thinking for health systems strengthening*. Geneva, Switzerland: Alliance for Health Policy and Systems Research.

Dick, B. 2009. *Vulnerability and most at risk: Towards a common framework*. Presentation, IYWG (Interagency Youth Working Group) Meeting on Young People Most-At-Risk for HIV/AIDS, Washington, DC, June 25.

DFID (UK Department for International Development). *Where we work*. http://www.dfid.gov.uk/Where-we-work/ (accessed June 23, 2010).

Dorenbaum, A., C. K. Cunningham, R. D. Gelber, M. Culnane, L. Mofenson, P. Britto, C. Rekacewicz, M. L. Newell, J. F. Delfraissy, B. Cunningham-Schrader, M. Mirochnick, and J. L. Sullivan. 2002. Two-dose intrapartum/newborn nevirapine and standard antiretroviral therapy to reduce perinatal HIV transmission: A randomized trial. *JAMA* 288(2):189–198.

DoS (U.S. Department of State). 2010a. *FY2011 Congressional budget justification volume 2—Foreign operations.* Washington, DC: DoS.

DoS. 2010b. *Implementation of the Global Health Initiative: Consultation document.* Washington, DC: DoS.

DoS OIG (U. S. Department of State and the Broadcasting Board of Governors Office of Inspector General). 2008. *Review of the Office of the U.S. Global AIDS Coordinator.* Report Number ISP-I-08-23. Washington, DC: DoS.

DoS OIG. 2009. *The exercise of chief of mission authority in managing the President's Emergency Plan for AIDS Relief overseas.* Report Number ISP-I-10-01. Washington, DC: DoS.

Dutta, A., and L. Fleisher. 2008. *Planning for sustainable HIV/AIDS services using the HAPSAT tool.* Presentation, Global Health Council Conference, Washington, DC, May 27.

Dybul, M. 2009. Lessons learned from PEPFAR. *J Acquir Immune Defic Syndr* 52(Suppl. 1):S12–S13.

Edgil, D. 2010. *The President's Emergency Plan for AIDS Relief: Public health evaluations.* Presentation, Public information-gathering session of the Committee on Planning the Assessment/Evaluation of HIV/AIDS Programs Implemented Under the U.S. Global Leadership Against HIV/AIDS, Tuberculosis, and Malaria Reauthorization Act of 2008, Washington, DC, January 7.

Emery, S., J. A. Neuhaus, A. N. Phillips, A. Babiker, C. J. Cohen, J. M. Gatell, P. M. Girard, B. Grund, M. Law, M. H. Losso, A. Palfreeman, and R. Wood. 2008. Major clinical outcomes in antiretroviral therapy (ART)-naive participants and in those not receiving ART at baseline in the SMART study. *J Infect Dis* 197(8):1133–1144.

Forsythe, S., J. Stover, and L. Bollinger. 2009. *The past, present and future of HIV/AIDS and resource allocation.* Working Paper No. 20. Washington, DC: aids2031.

Frenk, J. 2010. The global health system: Strengthening national health systems as the next step for global progress. *PLoS Med* 7(1):e1000089.

GAO (U.S. Government Accountability Office). 2004. *Global Health: U.S. AIDS Coordinator addressing some key challenges to expanding treatment, but others remain.* GAO-04-784. Washington, DC: GAO.

GAO. 2005. *Global HIV/AIDS epidemic: Selection of antiretroviral medications provided under U.S. emergency plan is limited.* GAO-05-133. Washington, DC: GAO.

GAO. 2006. *Global health: Spending requirement presents challenges for allocating prevention funding under the President's Emergency Plan for AIDS Relief.* GAO-06-395. Washington, DC: GAO.

GAO. 2008. *Global HIV/AIDS: A more country-based approach could improve allocation of PEPFAR funding.* GAO-08-480. Washington, DC: GAO.

GAO. 2009. *President's Emergency Plan for AIDS Relief: Partner selection and oversight follow accepted practices but would benefit from enhanced planning and accountability.* GAO-09-666. Washington, DC: GAO.

Garnett, G. P. 2002. An introduction to mathematical models in sexually transmitted disease epidemiology. *Sex Transm Infect* 78(1):7–12.

GFATM (The Global Fund to Fight AIDS, Tuberculosis and Malaria). 2009. *Global Fund ARV fact sheet: 1st December, 2009.* Geneva, Switzerland: GFTAM.

GFATM. 2010a. *Grant portfolio.* http://portfolio.theglobalfund.org/?lang=en (accessed June 23, 2010).

GFATM. 2010b. *The Global Fund 2010: Innovation and impact.* Geneva, Switzerland: GAFTM.

Girardi, E., G. Antonucci, P. Vanacore, M. Libanore, I. Errante, A. Matteelli, and G. Ippolito. 2000. Impact of combination antiretroviral therapy on the risk of tuberculosis among persons with HIV infection. *AIDS* 14(13):1985–1991.

Global HIV Prevention Working Group. 2010. *Key facts.* http://www.globalhivprevention.org/key_facts.html (accessed June 24, 2010).

Gouws, E., K. A. Stanecki, R. Lyerla, and P. D. Ghys. 2008. The epidemiology of HIV infection among young people aged 15–24 years in Southern Africa. *AIDS* 22(Suppl. 4):S5–S16.

Granich, R. M., C. F. Gilks, C. Dye, K. M. De Cock, and B. G. Williams. 2009. Universal voluntary HIV testing with immediate antiretroviral therapy as a strategy for elimination of HIV transmission: A mathematical model. *Lancet* 373(9657):48–57.

Granich, R., S. Crowley, M. Vitoria, Y. R. Lo, Y. Souteyrand, C. Dye, C. Gilks, T. Guerma, K. M. De Cock, and B. Williams. 2010. Highly active antiretroviral treatment for the prevention of HIV transmission. *J Int AIDS Soc* 13(1):1.

Gray, R. H., G. Kigozi, D. Serwadda, F. Makumbi, S. Watya, F. Nalugoda, N. Kiwanuka, L. H. Moulton, M. A. Chaudhary, M. Z. Chen, N. K. Sewankambo, F. Wabwire-Mangen, M. C. Bacon, C. F. Williams, P. Opendi, S. J. Reynolds, O. Laeyendecker, T. C. Quinn, and M. J. Wawer. 2007. Male circumcision for HIV prevention in men in Rakai, Uganda: A randomised trial. *Lancet* 369(9562):657–666.

Greene, J. C., V. J. Caracelli, and W. F. Graham. 1989. Toward a conceptual framework for mixed-method evaluation design. *Educ Eval Policy An* 11(3):255–274.

Gupta, R. K., A. Hill, A. W. Sawyer, A. Cozzi-Lepri, V. WYL, S. Yerly, V. Dias Lima, H. F. Günthard, C. Gilks, and D. Pillay. 2009. Virological monitoring and resistance to first-line HAART in adults infected with HIV-1 treated under WHO guidelines: Systematic review and meta-analysis. *Lancet Infect Dis* 9:409–417.

Hallett, T. B., B. Zaba, J. Todd, B. Lopman, W. Mwita, S. Biraro, S. Gregson, J. T. Boerma, and on behalf of the Alpha Network. 2008. Estimating incidence from prevalence in generalised HIV epidemics: Methods and validation. *PLoS Med* 5(4):e80.

Hallett, T. B., P. Ghys, T. Bärnighausen, P. Yan, G. P. Garnett. 2009. Errors in "BED"-derived estimates of HIV incidence will vary by place, time and age. *PLoS One* 4(5):e5720.

Hammer, S. 2010. *ART is great.* Presentation, 17th Conference on Retroviruses and Opportunistic Infections (CROI), San Francisco, CA, February 16–19.

Heaton, L. M., R. Komatsu, D. Low-Beer, T. B. Fowler, and P. O. Way. 2008. Estimating the number of HIV infections averted: An approach and issues. *Sex Transm Infect* 84(Suppl. 1):i92–i96.

Herbst, A. J., G. S. Cooke, T. Barnighausen, A. KanyKany, F. Tanser, and M. L. Newell. 2009. Adult mortality and antiretroviral treatment roll-out in rural Kwazulu-Natal, South Africa. *Bull World Health Organ* 87(10):754–762.

High-Level Forum. 2005. Paris declaration on aid effectiveness: Ownership, harmonization, alignment, results, and mutual accountability, Paris, France, February 28–March 2.

Holmes, C. 2009. *Using costing and modeling to improve treatment (and other) program planning.* Presentation, PEPFAR Annual Meeting with Track One Partners, Dar es Salaam, Tanzania, August 4.

Hussey, M. A., and J. P. Hughes. 2007. Design and analysis of stepped wedge cluster randomized trials. *Contemp Clin Trials* 28(2):182–191.

IEG World Bank (Independent Evaluation Group of The World Bank Group). 2009. Improving effectiveness and outcomes for the poor in health, nutrition, and population: An evaluation of World Bank Group support since 1997. Washington, DC: The World Bank.

IOM (Institute of Medicine). 2005. *Plan for a short-term evaluation of PEPFAR implementation.* Washington, DC: The National Academies Press.

IOM. 2006. *Preventing HIV infection among injecting drug users in high risk countries: An assessment of the evidence.* Washington, DC: The National Academies Press.

IOM. 2007. *PEPFAR implementation: Progress and promise.* Washington, DC: The National Academies Press.

IOM. 2008. *Design considerations for evaluating the impact of PEPFAR: Workshop summary.* Washington, DC: The National Academies Press.

Jahn, A., S. Floyd, A. C. Crampin, F. Mwaungulu, H. Mvula, F. Munthali, N. McGrath, J. Mwafilaso, V. Mwinuka, B. Mangongo, P. E. Fine, B. Zaba, and J. R. Glynn. 2008. Population-level effect of HIV on adult mortality and early evidence of reversal after introduction of antiretroviral therapy in Malawi. *Lancet* 371(9624):1603–1611.

Jemmott, J. B. I., L. S. Jemmott, A. O'Leary, Z. Ngwane, L. D. Icard, S. L. Bellamy, S. F. Jones, G. A. Heeren, J. C. Tyler, and M. B. Makiwane. (in press). School-based randomized controlled trial of an HIV/std risk-reduction intervention for South African adolescents. *Arch Pediatr Adolesc Med.*

Jewkes, R., M. Nduna, J. Levin, N. Jama, K. Dunkle, A. Puren, and N. Duvvury. 2008. Impact of stepping stones on incidence of HIV and HSV-2 and sexual behaviour in rural South Africa: Cluster randomised controlled trial. *BMJ* 337(337):a506.

JLICA (The Joint Learning Initiative on Children and HIV/AIDS). 2009. *Home truths: Facing the facts on children, AIDS, and poverty.* Boston, MA: JLICA.

Johansson, K. A., B. Robberstad, and O. F. Norheim. 2010. Further benefits by early start of HIV treatment in low income countries: Survival estimates of early versus deferred antiretroviral therapy. *AIDS Res Ther* 7(1):3.

Kalichman, S. C., L. C. Simbayi, R. Vermaak, D. Cain, G. Smith, J. Mthebu, and S. Jooste. 2008. Randomized trial of a community-based alcohol-related HIV risk-reduction intervention for men and women in Cape Town South Africa. *Ann Behav Med* 36(3):270–279.

Kates, J., E. Lief, and C. Avila. 2009. *Financing the response to AIDS in low- and middle-income countries: International assistance from the G8, European Commission and other donor governments in 2008.* Washington, DC: Kaiser Family Foundation and UNAIDS.

Kaur, G., and A. Singh. 2010. *The "see and treat" approach to cervical cancer.* http://www.thelancetstudent.com/2010/02/16/the-see-and-treat-approach-to-cervical-cancer/ (accessed February 16, 2010).

KFF (Kaiser Family Foundation). 2009. *The global HIV/AIDS epidemic: Fact sheet.* Washington, DC: KFF.

Kuhn, L., G. M. Aldrovandi, M. Sinkala, C. Kankasa, K. Semrau, M. Mwiya, P. Kasonde, N. Scott, C. Vwalika, J. Walter, M. Bulterys, W. Y. Tsai, and D. M. Thea. 2008. Effects of early, abrupt weaning on HIV-free survival of children in Zambia. *N Engl J Med* 359(2):130–141.

Kuhn, L., G. M. Aldrovandi, M. Sinkala, C. Kankasa, K. Semrau, P. Kasonde, M. Mwiya, W. Y. Tsai, and D. M. Thea. 2009. Differential effects of early weaning for HIV-free survival of children born to HIV-infected mothers by severity of maternal disease. *PLoS ONE* 4(6):e6059.

Lawn, S. D., A. D. Harries, X. Anglaret, L. Myer, and R. Wood. 2008. Early mortality among adults accessing antiretroviral treatment programmes in sub-Saharan Africa. *AIDS* 22(15):1897–1908.

Leeuw, F., and J. Vaessen. 2009. *Impact evaluations and development NONIE guidance on impact evaluation.* Washington, DC: NONIE (Network of Networks for Impact Evaluation).

Levine, W. C. 2010. *CDC's role in PEPFAR strategic information and public health evaluation.* Presentation, Public information-gathering session of the Committee on Planning the Assessment/Evaluation of HIV/AIDS Programs Implemented Under the U.S. Global Leadership Against HIV/AIDS, Tuberculosis, and Malaria Reauthorization Act of 2008, Washington, DC, January 7.

Lima, V. D., K. Johnston, R. S. Hogg, A. R. Levy, P. R. Harrigan, A. Anema, and J. S. Montaner. 2008. Expanded access to highly active antiretroviral therapy: A potentially powerful strategy to curb the growth of the HIV epidemic. *J Infect Dis* 198(1):59–67.

Marsh, P. 2009. Presentation, First Committee Meeting on Planning the Assessment/Evaluation of HIV/AIDS Programs Implemented Under the U.S. Global Leadership Against HIV/AIDS, Tuberculosis, and Malaria Reauthorization Act of 2008, Washington, DC, November 23.

MEASURE DHS (Demographic and Health Surveys). 2010. *HIV/AIDS survey indicators database.* http://www.measuredhs.com/hivdata/ (accessed April 14, 2010).

MEASURE Evaluation. 2007. *Monitoring and evaluation systems strengthening tool.* Chapel Hill, NC: MEASURE Evaluation.

MEASURE Evaluation. 2009. *Child status index a tool for assessing the well-being of orphans and vulnerable children—Manual.* Chapel Hill, NC: MEASURE Evaluation.

Mermin, J., W. Were, J. P. Ekwaru, D. Moore, R. Downing, P. Behumbiize, J. R. Lule, A. Coutinho, J. Tappero, and R. Bunnell. 2008. Mortality in HIV-infected Ugandan adults receiving antiretroviral treatment and survival of their HIV-uninfected children: A prospective cohort study. *Lancet* 371(9614):752–759.

Moloney-Kitts, M. 2009. *Update on the U.S. response to the global AIDS pandemic.* Presentation, Public information-gathering session of the Committee on Planning the Assessment/Evaluation of HIV/AIDS Programs Implemented Under the U.S. Global Leadership Against HIV/AIDS, Tuberculosis, and Malaria Reauthorization Act of 2008, Washington, DC, November 23.

Montaner, J. S., R. Hogg, E. Wood, T. Kerr, M. Tyndall, A. R. Levy, and P. R. Harrigan. 2006. The case for expanding access to highly active antiretroviral therapy to curb the growth of the HIV epidemic. *Lancet* 368(9534):531–536.

Murphy, G., and J. V. Parry. 2008. Assays for the detection of recent infections with human immunodeficiency virus type 1. *Euro Surveill* 13(36):18966.

Napierala-Mavedzenge, S., A. Doyle, and D. Ross. 2010. *HIV prevention in young people in sub-Saharan Africa: A systematic review.* London School of Hygiene & Tropical Medicine Health Policy Unit. London: London School of Hygiene & Tropical Medicine.

Newell, M. L., H. Coovadia, M. Cortina-Borja, N. Rollins, P. Gaillard, and F. Dabis. 2004. Mortality of infected and uninfected infants born to HIV-infected mothers in Africa: A pooled analysis. *Lancet* 364(9441):1236–1243.

Nyamukapa, C. A., S. Gregson, B. Lopman, S. Saito, H. J. Watts, R. Monasch, and M. C. Jukes. 2008. HIV-associated orphanhood and children's psychosocial distress: Theoretical framework tested with data from Zimbabwe. *Am J Public Health* 98(1):133–141.

OGAC (Office of the U.S. Global AIDS Coordinator). 2004. *The U.S. President's Emergency Plan for AIDS Relief: U.S. Five year global HIV/AIDS strategy.* Washington, DC: OGAC.

OGAC. 2006a. *Bringing hope: Supplying antiretroviral drugs for HIV/AIDS treatment. The President's Emergency Plan for AIDS Relief: Report on antiretroviral drugs for HIV/AIDS treatment.* Washington, DC: OGAC.

OGAC. 2006b. *Guidance for United States government in-country staff and implementing partners for a preventive care package for adults*- #1.* Washington, DC: OGAC.

OGAC. 2006c. *Guidance for United States government in-country staff and implementing partners for a preventive care package for children aged 0–14 years old born to HIV-infected mothers* - #1.* Washington, DC: OGAC.

OGAC. 2006d. *HIV/AIDS palliative care guidance #1 for the United States government in-country staff and implementing partners.* Washington, DC: OGAC.

OGAC. 2006e. *Orphans and other vulnerable children programming guidance for United States government in-country staff and implementing partners.* Washington, DC: OGAC.

OGAC. 2006f. *The President's Emergency Plan for AIDS Relief report on gender-based violence and HIV/AIDS.* Washington, DC: OGAC.

OGAC. 2006g. *The President's Emergency Plan for AIDS Relief: Report on food and nutrition for people living with HIV/AIDS.* Washington, DC: OGAC.

OGAC. 2008a. *The power of partnerships: The U.S. President's Emergency Plan for AIDS Relief. 2008 annual report to Congress.* Washington, DC: OGAC.

OGAC. 2008b. *The U.S. President's Emergency Plan for AIDS Relief (PEPFAR)—Fiscal Year 2008: PEPFAR operational plan.* Washington, DC: OGAC.

OGAC. 2009a. *Celebrating life: The U.S. President's Emergency Plan for AIDS Relief. 2009 annual report to Congress.* Washington, DC: OGAC.

OAGC. 2009b. *Guidance for PEPFAR partnership frameworks and partnership framework implementation plans. Version 2.0.* Washington, DC: OGAC.

OGAC. 2009c. *PEPFAR: State of the program area.* Washington, DC: OGAC.

OGAC. 2009d. *The President's Emergency Plan for AIDS Relief next generation indicators reference guidance. Version 1.1.* Washington, DC: OGAC.

OGAC. 2009e. *The President's Emergency Plan for AIDS Relief. FY2010 country operational guidance: Programmatic considerations.* Washington, DC: OGAC.

OGAC. 2009f. *The U.S. President's Emergency Plan for AIDS Relief (PEPFAR)—Fiscal year 2009: PEPFAR operational plan.* Washington DC: OGAC.

OGAC. 2009g. *The U.S. President's Emergency Plan for AIDS Relief: Five-year strategy.* Washington, DC: OGAC.

OGAC. 2009h. *The U.S. President's Emergency Plan for AIDS Relief: Five-year strategy. Annex: PEPFAR's contributions to the Global Health Initiative.* Washington, DC: OGAC.

OGAC. 2009i. *The U.S. President's Emergency Plan for AIDS Relief: Five-year strategy. Annex: PEPFAR and prevention, care, and treatment.* Washington, DC: OGAC.

OGAC. 2010. *The U.S. President's Emergency Plan for AIDS Relief: 2009 annual report to Congress on PEPFAR program results.* Washington, DC: OGAC.

OHCHR (Office of the High Commissioner for Human Rights). 2007. *Committee on the rights of the child: Sessions.*
http://www2.ohchr.org/english/bodies/crc/sessions.htm (accessed May 28, 2010).

PEPFAR (U.S. President's Emergency Plan for AIDS Relief). 2007. *About OGAC: Organizational chart.*
http://www.pepfar.gov/c22835.htm (accessed March 25, 2010).

PEPFAR. 2008a. *Data quality assessment tool (for auditing and capacity building).*
http://www.pepfar.gov/implementer_resources/data_quality/c20984.htm (accessed May 17, 2010).

PEPFAR. 2008b. *Premier global companies, U.S. government launch unprecedented partnership for an HIV-Free Generation. The U.S. President's Emergency Plan for AIDS Relief announces public-private partnership for global HIV prevention for youth.* HIV-Free Generation Press Release, December 5.
http://www.pepfar.gov/documents/organization/112564.pdf (accessed April 16, 2010).

PEPFAR. 2009a. *Draft agenda.* The United States President's Emergency Plan for AIDS Relief Annual Meeting—Optimizing the Response: Partnerships for Sustainability, Windhoek, Namibia, June 8–10.

PEPFAR. 2009b. *Technical support to Global Fund grants (updated September 2009).*
http://www.pepfar.gov/coop/boardmeetings/91395.htm (accessed June 14, 2010).

PEPFAR. 2009c. *Total number of individuals reached (on antiretroviral treatment FY2005–FY2008).*
http://www.pepfar.gov/about/tables/treatment/123461.htm (accessed March 9, 2010).

PEPFAR. 2010a. *Implementing agencies: Department of Commerce (DoC).*
http://www.pepfar.gov/agencies/c19398.htm (accessed June 15, 2010).

PEPFAR. 2010b. *Technical note on PEPFAR's reporting methodology: Results of USG Global Fund contributions.* http://www.pepfar.gov/2009results/ (accessed June 16, 2010).

PEPFAR. 2010c. *The U.S. President's Emergency Plan for AIDS Relief: Reports.*
http://www.pepfar.gov/progress/index.htm (accessed April 14, 2010).

PEPFAR and USAID (United States Agency for International Development). 2007. *Data quality assurance tool for program-level indicators.* Washington, DC: USAID.

PEPFAR Reauthorization Action Team. 2010. *Top 11 facts to know about PEPFAR.*
http://www.pepfar2.org/facts.html#top10 (accessed March 9, 2010).

Phillips, A., and J. van Oosterhout. 2010. DART points the way for HIV treatment programmes. *Lancet* 375(9709):96–98.

PMI (The President's Malaria Initiative). 2009. *Fast facts: The President's Malaria Initiative (PMI).* Washington, DC: PMI.

Resch, S., H. Wang, M. Kayode Ogungbemi, and G. Kombe. 2009. *Sustainability analysis of HIV/AIDS services in Nigeria.* Bethesda, MD: Health Systems 20/20 Project, Abt Associates Inc.

Rugg, D., G. Peersman, and M. Carael, eds. 2004. *Global advances in HIV/AIDS monitoring and evaluation: New directions for evaluation.* San Francisco, CA: Jossey-Bass.

Samb, B., T. Evans, M. Dybul, R. Atun, J. P. Moatti, S. Nishtar, A. Wright, F. Celletti, J. Hsu, J. Y. Kim, R. Brugha, A. Russell, and C. Etienne. 2009. An assessment of interactions between global health initiatives and country health systems. *Lancet* 373(9681):2137–2169.

Shaffer, N., M. McConnell, O. Bolu, D. Mbori-Ngacha, T. Creek, R. Ntumy, and L. Mazhani. 2004. Prevention of mother-to-child HIV transmission internationally. *Emerg Infect Dis* 10(11):2027–2028.

Shakarishvili, G. 2009 (unpublished). *Building on health systems frameworks for developing a common approach to health systems strengthening.* Paper presented at World Bank, the Global Fund and the GAVI Alliance Technical Workshop on Health Systems Strengthening, Washington, DC, June 25–27.

Stanton, B. F., X. Li, J. Kahihuata, A. M. Fitzgerald, S. Neumbo, G. Kanduuombe, I. B. Ricardo, J. S. Galbraith, N. Terreri, I. Guevara, H. Shipena, J. Strijdom, R. Clemens, and R. F. Zimba. 1998. Increased protected sex and abstinence among Namibian youth following a HIV risk-reduction intervention: A randomized, longitudinal study. *AIDS* 12(18):2473–2480.

Stanton, D. 2009. *Program guidance and updates: Report on TAB, SOPA.* Oral Presentation, The United States President's Emergency Plan for AIDS Relief Annual Meeting, United States Government Days Meeting, Windhoek, Namibia, June8.

Stover, J., B. Fidzani, B. C. Molomo, T. Moeti, and G. Musuka. 2008. Estimated HIV trends and program effects in Botswana. *PLoS ONE* 3(11):e3729.

UNAIDS (United Nations Joint Programme on HIV/AIDS). 2004. *"Three ones" key principles.* Conference paper 1, Washington consultation of April 4, 2004. Geneva, Switzerland: UNAIDS.

UNAIDS. 2006. *2006 report on the global AIDS epidemic.* Geneva, Switzerland: UNAIDS.

UNAIDS. 2008. *Report on the global AIDS epidemic 2008.* Geneva, Switzerland: UNAIDS.

UNAIDS. 2009a. *Operational plan for the UNAIDS action framework: Addressing women, girls, gender equality and HIV.* Geneva, Switzerland: UNAIDS.

UNAIDS. 2009b. *Spectrum 2009: Estimates and projections of national HIV/AIDS epidemics.* Presentation. http://data.unaids.org/pub/Presentation/2009/20090414_spectrum_2009_en.pdf (accessed June 22, 2010).

UNAIDS. 2010a. *Gender.* http://www.unaids.org/en/PolicyAndPractice/Gender/default.asp (accessed April 27, 2010).

UNAIDS. 2010b. *Key populations.* http://www.unaids.org/en/PolicyAndPractice/KeyPopulations/default.asp (accessed April 9, 2010).

UNAIDS, UNICEF, and USAID (United Nations Joint Programme on HIV/AIDS, United Nations Children's Fund, and United States Agency for International Development). 2002. *Children on the brink 2002: A joint report on orphan estimates and program strategies.* Washington, DC: UNAIDS/UNICEF/USAID.

UNAIDS, UNICEF, and USAID. 2004. *Children on the brink 2004: A joint report on new orphan estimates and a framework for action.* Washington, DC: UNAIDS/UNICEF/USAID.

UNAIDS and WHO (United Nations Joint Programme on HIV/AIDS and World Health Organization). 2009. *AIDS epidemic update: December 2009.* Geneva, Switzerland: UNAIDS.

UNAIDS MERG (United Nations Joint Programme on HIV/AIDS Monitoring & Evaluation Reference Group). 2010. *Guidance on developing terms of reference for HIV prevention evaluation.* Geneva, Switzerland: UNAIDS.

UNAIDS Reference Group on Estimates Modelling and Projections. 2002. Improved methods and assumptions for estimation of the HIV/AIDS epidemic and its impact: Recommendations of the UNAIDS Reference Group on Estimates, Modelling and Projections. *AIDS* 16(9):W1–W14.

UNAIDS Reference Group on Estimates Modelling and Projections. 2007. *Estimation of orphanhood due to HIV/AIDS and non-AIDS causes and the impact of intervention programmes.* Report of a meeting of the UNAIDS Reference Group on Estimates, Modelling, and Projections, Baltimore, July 12.

UNGASS (United Nations General Assembly Special Session). 2001. *Declaration of commitment on HIV/AIDS.* New York: United Nations.

UNICEF (United Nations Children's Fund). 2004. *The framework for the protection, care and support of orphans and vulnerable children living in a world with HIV and AIDS.* New York: UNICEF.

UNICEF. 2007. *Enhanced protection for children affected by AIDS. A companion paper to the framework for the protection, care and support of orphans and vulnerable children living in a world with HIV and AIDS.* New York: UNICEF.

UNICEF. 2009. *Children and AIDS: Fourth stocktaking report, 2009.* New York: UNICEF, United Nations Joint Programme on HIV/AIDS, World Health Organization, and United Nations Population Fund.

UNITAID and CHAI (UNITAID and Clinton Health Access Initiative). 2010. *Agreement for the procurement and supply of second-line ARV drugs for 2010.* Geneva, Switzerland: UNITAID.

UNITAID. 2010. *UNITAID: Mission.* http://www.unitaid.eu/en/UNITAID-Mission.html (accessed April 11, 2010).

United Nations. 1990. *Convention on the Rights of the Child.* New York: United Nations.

United Nation. 2003. *Monterrey Consensus on Financing for Development.* The final text of agreements and commitments adopted at the International Conference on Financing for Development, Monterrey, Mexico, 18–22 March 2002. New York: United Nations.

UNIFEM (United Nations Development Fund for Women). 2006. *Transforming the national AIDS response: Mainstreaming gender equality and women's human rights into the "Three Ones".* New York: UNIFEM.

United Nations General Assembly. 2006. *Political declaration on HIV/AIDS.* New York: United Nations.

United Nations Treaty Collection. 2010. *Convention on the Rights of the Child (status as of 14-04-2010).* http://treaties.un.org/Pages/ViewDetails.aspx?src=TREATY&mtdsg_no=IV-11&chapter=4&lang=en (accessed April 16, 2010).

USAID (United States Agency for International Development). 2000. *USAID/India: Life initiative leadership and investment in fighting an epidemic.* http://www.usaid.gov/press/releases/2000/fs20000079.htm (accessed May 6, 2010).

USAID. 2009a. *Food for peace.* http://www.usaid.gov/our_work/humanitarian_assistance/ffp/history.html (accessed May 28, 2010).

USAID. 2009b. *USAID's HIV/AIDS annual budget.* http://www.usaid.gov/our_work/global_health/aids/Funding/index.html (accessed May 6, 2010).

USAID and DoS. 2009 (United States Agency for International Development and U.S. Department of State). *Addressing water challenges in the developing world: A framework for action.* Washington, DC: Bureau of Economic Growth, Agriculture, and Trade, U.S. Agency for International Development and Bureau of Oceans, Environment, and Science, U.S. Department of State.

U.S. Census Bureau. 2009. *International data base: Population estimates and projections methodology.* Washington, DC: U.S. Census Bureau.

Violari, A., M. F. Cotton, D. M. Gibb, A. G. Babiker, J. Steyn, S. A. Madhi, P. Jean-Philippe, and J. A. McIntyre. 2008. Early antiretroviral therapy and mortality among HIV-infected infants. *N Engl J Med* 359(21):2233–2244.

von Linstow, M. L., V. Rosenfeldt, A. M. Lebech, M. Storgaard, T. Hornstrup, T. L. Katzenstein, G. Pedersen, T. Herlin, N. H. Valerius, and N. Weis. 2010. Prevention of mother-to-child transmission of HIV in Denmark, 1994–2008. *HIV Med* (Epub ahead of print).

WHO (World Health Organization). 1999. *Programming for adolescent health and development. Report of a WHO/UNFPA/UNICEF study group.* Geneva, Switzerland: WHO.

WHO. 2006a. *Guidelines on co-trimoxazole prophylaxis for HIV-related infections among children, adolescents and adults: Recommendations for a public health approach.* Geneva, Switzerland: WHO.

WHO. 2006b. *Patient monitoring guidelines for HIV care and antiretroviral therapy (ART).* Geneva, Switzerland: WHO.

WHO. 2006c. *Preventing HIV/AIDS in young people. A systematic review of the evidence from developing countries.* Geneva, Switzerland: WHO.

WHO. 2007a. *Everybody's business: Strengthening health systems to improve health outcomes. WHO's framework for action.* Geneva, Switzerland: WHO.

WHO. 2007b. *WHO case definitions of HIV for surveillance and revised clinical staging and immunological classification of HIV-related disease in adults and children.* Geneva, Switzerland: WHO.

WHO. 2008. *Essential prevention and care interventions for adults and adolescents living with HIV in resource-limited settings.* Geneva, Switzerland: WHO.

WHO. 2009a. *Rapid advice: Antiretroviral therapy for HIV infection in adults and adolescents.* Geneva, Switzerland: WHO.

WHO. 2009b. *Rapid advice: Use of antiretroviral drugs for treating pregnant women and preventing HIV infection in infants.* Geneva, Switzerland: WHO.

WHO. 2009c. *Rapid advice: WHO principles and recommendations on infant feeding in the context of HIV.* Geneva, Switzerland: WHO.

WHO. 2009d. *Women and health : Today's evidence tomorrow's agenda.* Geneva, Switzerland: WHO.

WHO. 2010. *Antiretroviral therapy for HIV infection in infants and children: Towards universal access. Executive summary of recommendations.* Preliminary version for program planning. Geneva, Switzerland: WHO.

WHO, UNAIDS, and UNICEF (World Health Organization, United Nations Joint Programme on HIV/AIDS, and United Nations Children's Fund). 2009. *Towards universal access: Scaling up priority HIV/AIDS interventions in the health sector. Progress report 2009.* Geneva, Switzerland: WHO.

WHO, UNFPA, and UNICEF (World Health Organization, United Nations Population Fund, and United Nations Children's Fund). 1997. *Action for adolescent health: Towards a common agenda. Recommendations from a joint study group.* Geneva, Switzerland: WHO.

Wood, E., T. Kerr, B. D. Marshall, K. Li, R. Zhang, R. S. Hogg, P. R. Harrigan, and J. S. Montaner. 2009. Longitudinal community plasma HIV-1 RNA concentrations and incidence of HIV-1 among injecting drug users: Prospective cohort study. *BMJ* 338:b1649.

World Bank. 2007. *The Africa Multi-country AIDS Program, 2000–2006: Results of the World Bank's response to a development crisis, edited by M. Görgens-Albino, N. Mohammad, D. Blankhart, and O. Odutolu.* Washington, DC: The World Bank.

World Bank. 2010. *Projects & Operations.* http://web.worldbank.org/WBSITE/EXTERNAL/PROJECTS/0,,menuPK:115635~pagePK:64020917~piPK:64021009~theSitePK:40941,00.html (accessed June 23, 2010).

Zachariah, R., A. D. Harries, M. Philips, L. Arnould, K. Sabapathy, D. P. O'Brien, C. Ferreyra, and S. Balkan. 2010. Antiretroviral therapy for HIV prevention: Many concerns and challenges, but are there ways forward in sub-Saharan Africa? *Trans R Soc Trop Med Hyg* 104(6): 387–391.

# Appendix A

# Statement of Task

As part of a two-step process, an ad hoc committee will undertake the first step to develop a plan for the assessment and evaluation of HIV/AIDS programs implemented under the U.S. Global Leadership Against HIV/AIDS, Tuberculosis, and Malaria Reauthorization Act of 2008 and issue a short report to the U.S. Congress on the plan's proposed design and budget by early 2010. The Institute of Medicine's Board on Global Health and the Board on Children, Youth, and Families will undertake this consensus study jointly. The second step will involve the actual conduct of the assessment and evaluation of the programs as a separate project after congressional review of the plan's proposed design and budget is completed.

(A) In its plan development, the committee will take cognizance of the following requirements for the congressionally mandated study, which must include:
(i) an assessment of the performance of United States-assisted global HIV/AIDS programs; and
(ii) an evaluation of the impact on health of prevention, treatment, and care efforts that are supported by United States funding, including multilateral and bilateral programs involving joint operations.

(B) Further the committee should provide:
(i) an assessment of progress toward prevention, treatment, and care targets;
(ii) an assessment of the effects on health systems, including on the financing and management of health systems and the quality of service delivery and staffing;
(iii) an assessment of efforts to address gender-specific aspects of HIV/AIDS, including gender related constraints to accessing services and addressing underlying social and economic vulnerabilities of women and men;
(iv) an evaluation of the impact of treatment and care programs on 5-year survival rates, drug adherence, and the emergence of drug resistance;
(v) an evaluation of the impact of prevention programs on HIV incidence in relevant population groups;
(vi) an evaluation of the impact on child health and welfare of interventions authorized under this Act on behalf of orphans and vulnerable children;
(vii) an evaluation of the impact of programs and activities authorized in this Act on child mortality; and
(viii) recommendations for improving the programs referred to in subparagraph (A)(i).

# Appendix B

# Committee and Staff Biographies

**Dr. Robert E. Black** *(Chair)* is the chairman of the Department of International Health and the Edgar Berman Professor in International Health, as well as the director of the Institute for International Programs of the Johns Hopkins Bloomberg School of Public Health. Dr. Black is trained in medicine, infectious diseases, and epidemiology. He has served as a medical epidemiologist at the U.S. Centers for Disease Control and Prevention and worked at institutions in Bangladesh and Peru on research related to childhood infectious diseases and nutritional problems. Dr. Black's current research includes field trials of vaccines, micronutrients, and other nutritional interventions, effectiveness studies of health programmes, and the evaluation of preventive and curative health service programmes in low- and middle-income countries. His other interests are related to the use of evidence in policy and programmes, including estimates of burden of disease and the development of research capacity. As a member of the Institute of Medicine (IOM) and advisory bodies of the World Health Organization, the International Vaccine Institute, and other international organizations, he assists with the development of policies intended to improve child health. He chairs the Child Health Epidemiology Reference Group and the Child Health and Nutrition Research Initiative. He currently has projects in Bangladesh, Ghana, India, Malawi, Mali, Peru, Tanzania, and Zanzibar. He has more than 450 scientific journal publications and is co-editor of the textbook "International Public Health." Dr. Black has served on four committees and the Board on International Health (now Global Health) of the IOM.

**Dr. Martha Ainsworth** is an Advisor to the World Bank's Independent Evaluation Group (IEG). An economist, she was formerly the coordinator for Health and Education Evaluation at IEG and was the lead author of IEG's 2009 evaluation of World Bank support for health, nutrition, and population since 1997 ("Improving Effectiveness and Outcomes for the Poor in Health, Nutrition, and Population") and of IEG's 2005 evaluation of World Bank support for HIV/AIDS ("Committing to Results: Improving the Effectiveness of HIV/AIDS Assistance"). She co-authored the IEG evaluation of support to primary education, "From Schooling Access to Learning Outcomes: An Unfinished Agenda," issued in 2006. Prior to joining IEG in 2001, she worked as a researcher in the Development Research Group and the Africa Technical Department of the World Bank. She has published research on the economics of HIV/AIDS prevention, the impact of HIV/AIDS mortality on children and the elderly, the potential demand for an AIDS vaccine, and fertility and family planning in Africa. She co-authored the World Bank Policy Research Report, "Confronting AIDS: Public Priorities in a Global Epidemic" (1997, 1999), and was on the core team of the World Development Report 1984 on population and development. She participated extensively in the piloting and implementation of the Bank's first Living Standards Measurement Surveys in the 1980s in Africa, and is an expert on household surveys. Prior to joining the World Bank, she taught secondary school in the U.S. Peace Corps in Chad and worked for the Peace Corps evaluation office. She holds an M.A. in international studies from Johns Hopkins University, specializing in economic development, public health, and African studies, and a Ph.D. in economics from Yale University.

**Dr. Pierre M. Barker** is professor of pediatrics at the University of North Carolina (UNC) at Chapel Hill. He is the senior technical director for the Developing Countries program and the director of Institute for Healthcare Improvement's (IHI) HIV/AIDS improvement projects in South Africa—currently active in six projects in five provinces covering rural/urban and adult/pediatric practices. He is a technical advisor to Project Fives Alive! and works at a variety of health care facilities, ranging from urban tertiary care to deep rural primary care. Ghana's Project Fives Alive! is sponsored by the Bill & Melinda Gates Foundation to reduce morbidity and mortality in children under five by 20 percent or more. Working first in the most-challenged regions of the north (Northern, Upper East, and Upper West), and then on a national scale, IHI and National Catholic Health Service work to improve health outcomes in this population while simultaneously enhancing—and permanently strengthening—the performance of the nation's faith-based and public health structures. Dr. Barker grew up in Durban, South Africa, and returned for 2004–2005 to South Africa, while on sabbatical leave, to establish IHI's projects in his native country. Outside of his IHI work, he is interested in pediatric lung diseases, is an attending physician for pediatric pulmonology, and leads health care system transformation projects for UNC Chapel Hill.

**Dr. Mary T. Bassett** is the director for the African Health Initiative at the Doris Duke Charitable Foundation. Before joining the Doris Duke Charitable Foundation, Dr. Bassett was the deputy commissioner for health promotion and disease prevention at the New York City Health Department. She joined the New York City Health Department in 2002 when she returned to New York City after many years based in Southern Africa. As deputy commissioner, Dr. Bassett oversaw a wide range of program areas, including non-communicable disease, school health and maternal and child health, as well as a network of District Public Health offices devoted to improving health conditions in low-income neighborhoods. Prior to joining the New York City Health Department, Dr. Bassett was the associate director of the Health Equity unit of the Rockefeller Foundation in Harare, Zimbabwe. As Associate Director, Dr. Bassett led the development of the Foundation's AIDS program, which included support of research in treatment and care. For 17 years, she worked at the University of Zimbabwe Medical School. Originally from New York City, Dr. Bassett received a B.A. from Radcliffe College and an M.D. from Columbia University. She completed her medical training at Harlem Hospital Center and received an M.P.H. from the University of Washington.

**Dr. Ronald Brookmeyer** is a professor of biostatistics at the University of California, Los Angeles School of Public Health. Prior to this, he was professor of biostatistics in the Department of Biostatistics at the Bloomberg School of Public Health at Johns Hopkins

University. Dr. Brookmeyer's research is at the interface of biostatistics and public health. A main theme of Dr. Brookmeyer's work concerns statistical and quantitative approaches for measuring the health of populations. Dr. Brookmeyer develops statistical methods and models for tracking and forecasting health and disease. He has worked extensively on the development of methods for tracking the course of the global HIV/AIDS epidemic. Dr. Brookmeyer developed the back-calculation method for disease forecasting and developed statistical approaches for biomarker-based methods for ascertaining HIV incidence rates in populations. He has also worked on issues of biosecurity, including epidemic models. His research interests in biostatistics include survival analysis, clinical trial design and analyses, and epidemiological and statistical methods for disease surveillance. Dr. Brookmeyer is currently the chair of the Statistics in Epidemiology Section of the American Statistical Association. He is a fellow of the American Association for the Advancement of Science and of the American Statistical Association. A member of the Institute of Medicine, he has served on six prior National Academies committees.

**Dr. David D. Celentano** is a professor and the chair of the Department of Epidemiology, with joint teaching appointments in the Departments of Health, Society, and Behavior and International Health at the Bloomberg School of Public Health at Johns Hopkins University, as well as in the School of Medicine. His research integrates behavioral science theory and research with epidemiology, in the study of behavioral and social epidemiology. While originally trained in a chronic disease paradigm (alcoholism and cancer control), he began his research in HIV/AIDS and sexually transmitted diseases (STDs) in the early 1980s. In this regard, he has worked on some of the major cohort studies (ALIVE, MACS) in HIV epidemiology, as well as conducted intervention research in the United States for heterosexual men and women, injection drug users, and young men who have sex with men. He turned to international research in 1990, when he began a long-term collaboration with Chiang Mai University in northern Thailand. He and his collaborators have demonstrated that a behavioral intervention with young men (military conscripts) leads to a seven-fold reduction in incident STDs and halving the HIV incidence rate. In addition, the role of STDs and alcohol use on HIV acquisition has been shown through his research. More recently, his group has conducted a prospective study of hormonal contraception in relation to HIV seroconversion and human papillomavirus (HPV) incidence, a study with significant family planning policy and health implications. Today, he is the principal investigator of four studies supported by the National Institutes of Health in Thailand, focusing on interventions to influence the association between opiate use, methamphetamine use, and other drugs on HIV. He is the author of over 450 peer-reviewed articles. He is co-editor of "Public Health Aspects of HIV/AIDS in Low and Middle Income Countries: Epidemiology, Prevention and Care" (Springer, 2008). Dr. Celentano has served on three prior Institute of Medicine committees.

**Dr. Angela Díaz** is the Jean C. and James W. Crystal Professor of Pediatrics and Community and Preventive Medicine at Mount Sinai School of Medicine. After earning her M.D. in 1981 at Columbia University College of Physicians and Surgeons, she completed her post-doctoral training at the Mount Sinai School of Medicine in 1985 and subsequently received a M.P.H. from Harvard University. Dr. Díaz is the director of the Mount Sinai Adolescent Health Center, a unique program that provides comprehensive, integrated, and interdisciplinary primary care, reproductive health, mental health, and health education services to teens. Under her leadership, the Center has become the largest adolescent specific health center in the U.S., seeing thousands of teens every year—for free. She is the president of the Board of Trustees of the Children's Aid Society of New York. Dr. Díaz has been a White House fellow, a member of the Food and Drug Administration Pediatric Advisory Committee, a member of the National Institutes of Health (NIH) State of the Science Conference on Preventing Violence and Related Health Risk Social Behaviors in Adolescents. She serves on an advisory panel for the NIH Reproductive Sciences Branch. She reviews grants for the NIH Institute of Child Health and Human Development Biobehavioral and Behavioral Sciences Committee, the NIH Partners in Research Program, the NIH Institute of Dental and Craniofacial Research, and the National Institute on Drug Abuse. The NIH has awarded several major grants to Dr. Díaz and her research team at the Mount Sinai Adolescent Health Center. In 2003, she chaired the National Advisory Committee on Children and Terrorism for Health and Human Services. In 2008, she was elected as a member of the Institute of Medicine (IOM) of the National Academy of Sciences. Dr. Díaz is active in public policy and advocacy in the United States and has conducted many international health projects in Asia, Central and South America, Europe, and Africa. She is a frequent speaker at conferences throughout the country and around the world. She has served on one prior IOM committee, and is currently a member of the IOM and National Research Council's Board on Children, Youth, and Families.

**Dr. Loretta Sweet Jemmott** is the van Ameringen Professor in Psychiatric Mental Health Nursing and the director of the Center for Health Equity Research at the University of Pennsylvania School of Nursing. She is one of the nation's foremost researchers in the field of HIV/AIDS prevention, with a consistent track record of evidenced-based HIV risk-reduction interventions. Dr. Jemmott, along with her research team, has received more than $100 million in federal funding devoted to designing and evaluating a series of outcome-based, theory-driven, culturally competent HIV sexual risk-reduction randomized controlled behavioral intervention trials with various populations, including African Americans, Latinos, Jamaicans, and South African adolescents, women, men, and families aimed at increasing safer sex behaviors. These trials have demonstrated remarkable success in reducing HIV risk associated behaviors while reducing the incidence of sexually transmitted diseases (STDs). To date, four of her evidenced-based interventions have been designated by the U.S. Centers for Disease Control and Prevention for national dissemination and have been translated into ongoing programs used both nationally and internationally by community-based organizations, schools, and clinics in high-risk urban areas. She has also worked extensively in South Africa and Botswana to help mitigate the magnitude of HIV/AIDS. Currently she is the co-investigator on four international NIH-funded randomized control trials (RCTs). In Botswana, she is the co-investigator on a National Institute of Child Health and Human Development (NICHD) funded HIV prevention research capacity building grant in partnership with the University of Pennsylvania and the University of Botswana. She is also a co-investigator on two NIH funded RCTs focusing on adolescents and adult men, and a HIV prevention study focusing on Jamaican mothers and their daughters. She recently received funding as Principal Investigator from NICHD for a RCT barbershop-based HIV/STD risk reduction for African American young men. Since her induction into the Institute of Medicine in 1999, she has served on two committees related to HIV and STD prevention.

**Jennifer Kates** is a vice president and the director of Global Health Policy and HIV at the Kaiser Family Foundation, where she oversees policy analysis and research focused on the domestic and global HIV epidemics. She has been working on HIV policy issues for 20 years and is a recognized expert in the field. In addition, Ms. Kates oversees the Foundation's broader global health policy projects and research, which provide timely policy analysis and data on the U.S. government's role in global health. Prior to joining the Foundation in 1998, Ms. Kates was a senior associate with The Lewin Group, a health care consulting firm, where she focused on HIV policy, strategic planning/health systems analysis, and health care for vulnerable populations. She previously worked at Princeton University, where she served as the director of the Lesbian, Gay, and Bisexual Concerns Office, and was also the coordinator of the University's Alcohol and Other Drugs Peer Education Program. Ms. Kates received her M.P.A. from Princeton University's Woodrow Wilson School of Public and International Affairs, and a B.A. in political science from Dartmouth College. She also holds a M.A. in political science from the University of Massachusetts. Currently, she is pursuing a Ph.D. in public policy at George Washington University, where she is also a lecturer.

**Dr. Ann Kurth** is a professor and the director of Global Health Initiatives at the College of Nursing at New York University (NYU). Prior to joining the NYU College of Nursing, Dr. Kurth was jointly appointed in the University of Washington (UW) School of Nursing and the UW Department of Global Health, where she maintains affiliate appointments. Dr. Kurth's research interests include behavioral epidemiology and the development of tools to improve HIV and other sexually transmitted infection prevention, screening, and care. Her research evaluates informatics as well as provider-delivered approaches in studies conducted in the United States and internationally. She is principal investigator of National Institutes of Health (NIH) and Gates Foundation-funded studies in Kenya, including a community-enrolled heterosexual couples' cohort and a randomized trial of a computerized counseling tool to promote positive prevention and antiretroviral therapy adherence. Other current studies include an NIH Challenge grant to test the real-world effectiveness of a Spanish-language intervention for Latinos living with HIV in New York City. She is co-investigator or consultant on other studies underway in the United States, Uganda, Kenya, India, and Peru. Dr. Kurth founded one of the first HIV care clinics in the Midwest, and has served as president of the Association of Nurses in AIDS Care. She edited one of the first books published on HIV in women (1993) and reviews for a number of journals including serving as an editorial board member for *STD*. She was a founding member of the UW Center for AIDS Research (CFAR) behavioral core, and currently is an executive committee member of the NYU CFAR. She received a Ph.D. in epidemiology from the University of Washington, an M.S.N., R.N., and C.N.M. in nurse-midwifery from Yale University, an M.P.H. in population and family health from Columbia University, and a B.A. with high distinction (African Studies minor) from Princeton University.

**Dr. Dora Mbanya** is a professor of hematology in the Faculty of Medicine and Biomedical Sciences at the University of Yaoundé I, and a consultant hematologist and chief of the Hematology and Transfusion Service at the University Teaching Hospital in Yaoundé, Cameroon. She sees a cohort of about 1,500 HIV-infected persons in her clinic, with about a thousand on antiretroviral therapy. From 2007 to 2009, she participated in a study sponsored by the National Institutes of Health on the molecular determinants of neuroAIDS in Cameroon. In 1998, she was awarded a grant to evaluate the knowledge, attitudes, and practices of nurses toward HIV/AIDS patients in a rural hospital of Cameroon. She has served in a number of workshops sponsored by the World Health Organization (WHO). Dr. Mbanya was the chair of the WHO training workshops on the clinical use of blood and blood products in Namibia and Ethiopia. Dr. Mbanya also worked on the WHO-sponsored evaluation of the pharmaceutical management of HIV/AIDS in Cameroon and was recently (July 2009) jointly accredited as a regional laboratory assessor by the WHO African Regional branch, in collaboration with the U.S. Centers for Disease Control and Prevention and A Global Healthcare Public Foundation. She is currently the national president of the Society for Women and AIDS in Africa, where she participates in reaching the community at various levels in an attempt to impact their lives positively. She has been an active member of the Cameroon Medical Women's Association where she has held several posts of responsibility. Dr. Mbanya received her M.D. from the University Center for Health Sciences, Yaoundé, Cameroon, a Diplôme Universitaire in transfusion medicine from the University of Abidjan in Côte d'Ivoire, and a Ph.D. in hematology from the University of Newcastle Upon Tyne, United Kingdom.

**Dr. Affette McCaw-Binns** is a professor of reproductive health epidemiology in the Department of Community Health and Psychiatry at the University of the West Indies, Mona, in Kingston, Jamaica. Her research is concerned with the epidemiology of perinatal and maternal mortality in the Caribbean, as well as antenatal and perinatal care in that region. She recently published on "Integrating Research into Policy and Programmes: Examples from the Jamaican Experience" and evaluated the World Health Organization (WHO) antenatal care trial. She is a member of the WHO's Maternal and Perinatal Health Topic Advisory Sub-Group on Classification System for Causes of Maternal Mortality and Morbidity. In 2009, she was awarded the University of the West Indies: Vice Chancellor's Award for Excellence for all-round excellent performance in research accomplishments and contribution to public service. Professor McCaw-Binns received her Ph.D. in perinatal epidemiology from the University of Bristol in England. She served on two Institute of Medicine committees including the Committee on the President's Emergency Plan for AIDS Relief Implementation Evaluation.

**Dr. Geeta Rao Gupta** is a senior fellow at the Bill & Melinda Gates Foundation Global Development Program. She provides advice to the president and leadership of the Global Development Program on their strategies and offers insight on managing projects to achieve the greatest impact. She advises the program on learning from those it aims to serve, and offers guidance on a range of cross-cutting issues and projects. Prior to joining the foundation, Dr. Rao Gupta was president of the International Center for Research on Women (ICRW), a position she assumed in 1997 after serving in a variety of roles, including consultant, researcher, and officer. As president of ICRW, Dr. Rao Gupta was internationally recognized for her expertise on gender and development issues, including women's health, economic empowerment, poverty alleviation, and gender equality. She is the recipient of numerous awards, including Harvard University's 2006 Anne Roe Award and the 2007 *Washington Business Journal's* "Women Who Mean Business" Award. Dr. Rao Gupta also serves on the Steering Committee of aids2031, an international initiative commissioned by the United Nations Joint Programme on HIV/AIDS, United States Agency for International Development's Advisory Committee for Voluntary Foreign Aid, and the boards of the Moriah Fund, the Nike Foundation, the MAC AIDS Fund and the Rural Development Institute. Dr. Rao Gupta has her B.A., M.A., and M.Phil. in psychology from the University of Delhi, and a Ph.D. in philosophy from Bangalore University in India.

**Dr. Douglas D. Richman** is a professor of pathology and medicine at the University of California, San Diego (UCSD) and the Florence Seeley Riford Chair in AIDS Research. He is the director of the Center for AIDS Research at UCSD and staff physician at the VA San Diego Healthcare System. He trained as an infectious disease physician and medical virologist at Stanford, the National Institutes of Health (NIH), and Harvard before joining the faculty at UCSD in 1976. He has focused his investigation on HIV disease and pathogenesis for the past 20 years. His laboratory was the first to identify HIV drug resistance. The lab joined two others in identifying latently infected CD4 cells as the obstacle to eradication of HIV with potent antiretroviral therapy. Recently his lab described the dynamics of the neutralizing antibody response to HIV and the rapidity of viral escape and evolution in response to this selective pressure. Dr. Richman has authored over 580 scientific publications. He is also a co-editor of "Clinical Virology," a state-of-the-art clinical reference book, and editor of "Antiviral Drug Resistance." Dr. Richman has served as a consultant to the NIH, the Veterans Administration, the World Health Organization, and the State of California, and has been honored with an NIH Merit Award and the Howard M. Temin Award for Clinical Science and Clinical Excellence in the Fight Against HIV/AIDS. He served on the Institute of Medicine Committee for Examining the Probable Consequences of Alternative Patterns of Widespread Antiretroviral Drug Use in Resource-Constrained Settings.

**Dr. Deborah L. Rugg** is the chief of the Monitoring and Evaluation Division at UNAIDS. Prior to joining UNAIDS, Dr. Rugg was the associate director for Monitoring and Evaluation for the Global AIDS Program of the U.S. Centers for Disease Control and Prevention in Atlanta. She was also an associate adjunct professor at Emory University School of Public Health. She was an assistant professor of health psychology at the University of California, San Francisco School of Medicine and San Diego State University School of Public Health for five years prior to joining the U.S. Centers for Disease Control and Prevention in 1987 as an Epidemic Intelligence Service Officer in the Division of HIV/STD Prevention. She has authored or coauthored more than 64 peer-reviewed publications and 27 major agency reports and publications, primarily in the areas of evaluation methodology, HIV prevention with adolescents, and HIV counseling and testing. She has a B.A. from the University of Wisconsin in physiological psychology, an M.A. from San Diego State University in experimental psychology, and a Ph.D. from the University of California, San Francisco School of Medicine in health psychology. Dr. Rugg served on the National Research Council Panel on Data and Research Priorities for Arresting AIDS in Sub-Saharan Africa.

**Dr. Dawn K. Smith** is a medical epidemiologist in the Division of HIV/AIDS Prevention at the U.S. Centers for Disease Control and Prevention (CDC), where she coordinates planning for potential domestic implementation of biomedical interventions to reduce HIV transmission (e.g., microbicides, pre-exposure prophylaxis) and serves as acting associate chief for science in the Epidemiology Branch. Dr. Smith began her career at CDC coordinating the HER Study, a multi-site longitudinal study of the effects of HIV-infection on women and collaborating with the National Institute of Allergy and Infectious Diseases (NIAID)-funded women's HIV cohort study, the WIHS. She then led the development of CDC guidelines for the use of non-occupational post-exposure prophylaxis and led the writing of a 5-year microbicide research agenda for the agency. She spent four years as the associate director for HIV research at the CDC field station in Botswana where she established clinical trial infrastructure with integrated sociobehavioral research and initiated PrEP trials. She maintains a strong research interest in the intersections of race, ethnicity, social class, injection drug use, and the HIV epidemic. Dr. Smith has served on scientific committees and review panels for NIAID, the Office of AIDS Research, and the National Institute on Drug Abuse. Dr. Smith received her M.D. from the University of Massachusetts Medical School and went on to complete an M.P.H. in public health policy and international health and an M.S. in clinical research design and statistical analysis at the University of Michigan. A family physician, Dr. Smith has practiced in varied settings, providing medical care in a Native American community; in an urban clinic with Hispanic, Vietnamese, and African-American families; and to HIV infected women at Grady Hospital in Atlanta.

**Dr. Sally K. Stansfield** is the executive secretary of the Health Metrics Network (HMN), responsible for managing the technical and financial contributions of HMN partners to accelerate reform of health information systems for improved health outcomes on behalf of the Network and its host, the World health Organization. Prior to 2006, Dr. Stansfield was the associate director for Global Health Strategies of the Bill & Melinda Gates Foundation. She draws upon more than 30 years of clinical and public health practice, with experience in research agencies, universities, governments, non-governmental organizations, and multilateral agencies. Dr. Stansfield's areas of expertise include public health research, policy, strategic planning, program design and development, evaluation, and the development of health information systems. She has designed and managed programs for the U.S. Centers for Disease Control and Prevention, the U.S. Agency for International Development, and Canada's International Development Research Centre, and has advised governments in Bangladesh, Cambodia, Ethiopia, Malawi, and the Democratic Republic of the Congo (among other countries, primarily in Asia and Africa). Her many awards include the Alpha Omega Alpha medical honorary, the International College of Surgeons Award for Scholarship, the Public Health Service Distinguished Service Commendation, a Fulbright Fellowship, and the Yale Tercentennial Medal.

**Dr. Jane Waldfogel** is a professor of social work and public affairs at Columbia University School of Social Work and a visiting professor at the Centre for Analysis of Social Exclusion at the London School of Economics. During the 2008–2009 academic year, she was the Marion Cabot Putnam Memorial Fellow at the Radcliffe Institute for Advanced Study at Harvard University where she was writing a book about Britain's war on poverty. She has written extensively on the impact of public policies on child and family well-being. Her books include "Steady Gains and Stalled Progress: Inequality and the Black-White Test Score Gap" (Russell Sage Foundation, 2008), "What Children Need" (Harvard University Press, 2006), "Securing the Future: Investing in Children from Birth to College" (Russell Sage Foundation, 2000), and "The Future of Child Protection: How to Break the Cycle of Abuse and Neglect" (Harvard University Press, 1998). Her current research includes studies related to work-family policies, poverty, social mobility, and income-related gaps in school readiness. Dr. Waldfogel received her Ph.D. in public policy from the Kennedy School of Government at Harvard University and an M.Ed. from the Harvard Graduate School of Education. She has served on one prior Institute of Medicine (IOM)-National Research Council (NRC) committee and is currently serving on the joint IOM-NRC Committee on Strengthening Benefit-Cost Methodology for the Evaluation of Early Childhood Interventions.

**Dr. Kathryn Whetten** is an associate professor of public policy, nursing, and community and family medicine studies at Duke University. She is the director of the Center for Health Policy-Health Inequities Program, as well as the research director for the Hart Fellows Program. Whetten assisted in the creation of Duke's Global Health Institute (DGHI) of which she is a member. Dr. Whetten's research focuses on evaluating and creating models of health care for chronically ill individuals. The target audience for her research is health policy analysts and decision makers, administrators, and clinicians. Dr. Whetten's area of study involves the identification of barriers to care, the creation of models of care that reduce barriers to care in a changing financial environment, the evaluation of such models, and engaging in the policy debate. Evaluation includes econometric models examining cost, health outcomes, utilization of health and human services, and satisfaction on the part of the patient and the provider. Much of Dr. Whetten's current research focuses on two of the most difficult populations to serve: those living with HIV, mental health, and/or substance disorders living around the world; and children who have been orphaned or abandoned. Dr. Whetten has lead more than 15 federally-funded research grants and is the author of two books and more than 50 peer reviewed articles. Currently Dr. Whetten and her intervention, service, and research team have research projects that address issues surrounding HIV/AIDS, mental health, substance abuse, being orphaned, social justice, and poverty in the U.S. Deep South, Tanzania, Kenya, Ethiopia, India (including Nagaland), Cambodia, Malawi, Cameroon, and Russia. A few of the research projects are: "Positive Outcomes for Children Orphaned by AIDS," "Coping with HIV/AIDS in Tanzania," "Integrative Treatment Model for Substance Abusing Women in Russia," and the "North Carolina HIV/AIDS Training Network," as well as collaborations with DGHI. Dr. Whetten received her Ph.D. in health policy research at the University of North Carolina, Chapel Hill.

**Dr. Catherine M. Wilfert** graduated with distinction from Stanford College in 1958 and then attended Harvard Medical School. After completion of her residency at North Carolina Baptist Hospital, she returned to Boston to continue to work in pediatrics and medicine. In 1971, she came to Duke University School of Medicine, where she achieved the rank of division chief of Pediatric Infectious Diseases and Professor in the Department of Pediatrics (1976–1994) and professor in the Department of Microbiology and Immunology. In 1996, she left Duke to become the scientific director of the Elizabeth Glaser Pediatric AIDS Foundation. Dr. Wilfert's work since the onset of AIDS has primarily been focused on the eradication of pediatric AIDS, and she is considered a seminal investigator in the field. She guided the National Institutes of Health AIDS Clinical Trial Group when the efficacy of using doses of zidovudine to reduce the incidence of mother-to-child transmission of HIV was accomplished. Mother-to-child transmission of HIV in the United States is estimated to be reduced to fewer than 200 cases per year. Dr. Wilfert now works to reduce mother-to-child transmission of AIDS in developing countries around the world. Dr. Wilfert has been on the editorial board of numerous publications and has served as a consultant for private companies, as well as U.S. and state governments. She is the recipient of many awards, including the 1997 Award of Recognition for Outstanding Contributions to Advancing the Prevention of Perinatal Transmission at A Global Strategies Conference for the Prevention of Mothers-to-Infants HIV Transmission. She also received a Lifetime Achievement Award in HIV from the Third International Meeting on HIV in India in 2001, and was given the Distinguished Award of Honor for Love of Humanity Especially in the Third World from the Cameroon Baptist Convention on Occasion of its 50th Anniversary Celebration in 2004. She was inducted to the Institute of Medicine (IOM) in 1999. Dr. Wilfert has served on five prior IOM committees and on the IOM Roundtable for the Development of Drugs and Vaccines Against AIDS.

## IOM STAFF

**Kimberly A. Scott** joined the Institute of Medicine's (IOM) Board on Global Health in September 2005 as a senior program officer. She has worked on several studies and activities including the Committee for the Evaluation of the President's Emergency Plan for AIDS Relief Implementation; Planning Committee on Preventing Violence in Low- and Middle-Income Countries; Committee on the Assessment of the Role of Intermittent Preventive Treatment for Malaria in Infants; Committee on Depression, Parenting Practices and the Health Development of Children; and the Committee on Achieving Global Sustainable Surveillance for Zoonotic Diseases. She is currently the study director for the PEPFAR Impact Evaluation. Prior to IOM, she was an analyst on the health care team at the U.S. Government Accountability Office. Before returning to graduate school, she coordinated programs at Duke University's Center for Health Policy, Law, and Management aimed at integrating mental health services into the continuum of care for people living with and affected by HIV/AIDS in 54 counties in North Carolina. For six years, she served as the Executive Director of a Ryan White-funded HIV/AIDS consortium, developing a comprehensive ambulatory care system for 21 mostly rural counties in North Carolina. Previous NC health-related committee service includes a number of advisory committees to the Governor of North Carolina and to the Secretary of NC DHHS for programmatic and policy issues related HIV care, prevention, and treatment. As an Echols Scholar, she received her B.A. in psychology from the University of Virginia. She received a M.S.P.H., with a concentration in health policy analysis, from the University of North Carolina, Chapel Hill.

**Dr. Bridget B. Kelly** is a program officer with the Institute of Medicine's Board on Global Health, where in addition to working on the PEPFAR Impact Evaluation she is the Study Director for the Committee on Preventing the Global Epidemic of Cardiovascular Disease: Meeting the Challenges in Developing Countries. She first came to the National Academies as a Christine Mirzayan Science and Technology Policy Graduate Fellow. Prior to joining the Board on Global Health, she worked in the Board on Children, Youth, and Families as staff for the Committee on the Prevention of Mental Disorders and Substance Abuse Among Children, Youth, and Young Adults, the Committee on Depression, Parenting Practices, and the Healthy Development of Children, and the Committee on Strengthening Benefit-Cost Methodology for the Evaluation of Early Childhood Interventions. She received her B.A. from Williams College and completed an M.D. and a Ph.D. in Neurobiology as part of the Medical Scientist Training Program at Duke University. In addition to her background in science and health, she has more than 10 years of experience in grassroots nonprofit arts administration.

**Ijeoma Emenanjo** is a senior program associate with the Board on African Science Academy Development. In this capacity, Ijeoma has spent the five years working on the Board on African Science Academy Development where he is primarily mentoring the staff at the National Academy of Nigeria on conducting convening activities and consensus studies. Ijeoma has also served as a Research Associate with the Board on Global Health for the Committee on the Assessment of the Role of Intermittent Preventive Treatment for Malaria in Infants. Before coming to the Academies in 2004, he worked on policy implementation issues such as HIV/AIDS prevention policy and electoral administration in Anglophone and Francophone West Africa. Prior to his transition into international policy work, Ijeoma was a polymeric materials engineer at the U.S. Army Research Lab in Adelphi, MD, and at the National Institutes of Standards and Technology's (Building and Fire Research Lab). Ijeoma received his B.S. in Chemical Engineering with a minor in economics from Howard University, and his M.P.P. from the University of Maryland, Baltimore County.

**Mila C. González** is a research associate with the Institute of Medicine's (IOM) Board on Global Health where she has served as research staff for the Committee on the Assessment of the Role of Intermittent Preventive Treatment for Malaria in Infants and the Committee on Achieving Sustainable Global Capacity for Surveillance and Response to Emerging Diseases of Zoonotic Origin. Before coming to the IOM in 2007, she worked as a clinical research assistant of a study evaluating the effects that exposure to violence has on young mothers with preschool-age children at the Children's National Medical Center Research Institute in Washington, DC. She received an M.P.H. in global health promotion from The George Washington University School of Public Health and Health Services and a B.S. in physiology and neurobiology from the University of Maryland, College Park.

**Kate Meck** is a research assistant with the Institute of Medicine's (IOM) Board on Global Health. She previously worked with the Committee on The U.S. Commitment to Global Health, the sequel to *America's Vital Interest in Global Health* (1997). Prior to joining the IOM, Kate was a program development intern at AYUDA, Inc., an international non-governmental organization that provides diabetes education in Latin America. She has worked extensively with international health programs in South Asia, Africa, and Latin America. Kate received a B.A. in International Relations, with minors in Economics and Spanish & Latin American Studies, from American University in 2007, and is currently pursuing an M.P.H. in global health design, monitoring, and evaluation at The George Washington University School of Public Health and Health Services.

**Kristen Danforth** is a senior program assistant with the Institute of Medicine's Board on Global Health, who recently completed work on her first study with the release of the report *Promoting Cardiovascular Health in the Developing World: A Critical Challenge to Achieve Global Health* (2010). She received her B.S. in International Health from Georgetown University in 2008, and is currently pursuing an M.P.H. at the Bloomberg School of Public Health at Johns Hopkins University.

**Dr. Carmen Cecilia Mundaca** is serving as an intern with the Institute of Medicine's Board on Global Health. Before traveling to the United States, she was employed as the Head of the Surveillance Center of the Emerging Infections Program in the United States Naval Medical Research Center Detachment in Lima, Peru. In that role Dr. Mundaca lead the successful implementation of a technology-based disease surveillance system (i.e., Alerta) at sites across the nation and initiated the broad adoption of Alerta in five other countries in South America. Alerta is a partnership involving the Peruvian Navy and the U.S. Navy; and provided the mechanism for reporting of 45 diseases/syndromes via a telephone or a computer with Internet access. She also led the collaborative syndromic surveillance pilot implementation in the Peruvian Ministry of

Health. Dr. Mundaca was part of the Early Warning Outbreak Recognition System (EWORS) Working Group and participated in several studies including a field visit to evaluate the performance of the system in Lao PDR. She obtained her M.D. from San Marcos University, Lima, Peru, and her M.P.H. degree from the Uniformed Services University of the Health Sciences, Bethesda, MD, where she is currently pursuing her Dr.P.H. degree. Her dissertation work will be focused on developing a framework that will serve as a guideline for the implementation of disease surveillance systems in developing countries. She plans to capitalize on the knowledge and experience gained on this project to contribute on developing her thesis work. Dr. Mundaca successfully completed a Certificate in Emerging Infectious Disease Epidemiology at the University of Iowa.

**Wendy E. Keenan** is a program associate with the Institute of Medicine's Board on Children, Youth, and Families. She helps organize planning meetings and workshops that cover current issues related to children, youth, and families as well as provides administrative and research support to the Board's various program committees. Wendy has been on the National Academies' staff for 10 years and worked on studies for both the Institute of Medicine and the National Research Council. As a senior program assistant, she worked with the National Research Council's Board on Behavioral, Cognitive, and Sensory Sciences. Prior to joining the National Academies, Wendy taught English as a second language for Washington, DC, public schools. She received a B.A. in sociology from The Pennsylvania State University and took graduate courses in liberal studies from Georgetown University.

**Julie Wiltshire** is a financial officer with the Institute of Medicine. Prior to joining the Institute of Medicine in 2004, she worked at Ernst & Young, LLP, as a financial auditor. She received a B.S. in accounting from Salisbury University.

**Rosemary Chalk** is the Director of the Board on Children, Youth, and Families, a joint effort of the Institute of Medicine and the National Research Council. She is a policy analyst who has been a study director at the National Academies since 1987. She has directed or served as a senior staff member for over a dozen studies in the Institute of Medicine and the National Research Council, including studies on vaccine finance, the public health infrastructure for immunization, family violence, child abuse and neglect, research ethics and misconduct in science, and education finance. From 2000 to 2003, she also directed a research project on the development of child well-being indicators for the child welfare system at Child Trends in Washington, DC. She has previously served as a consultant for science and society research projects at the Harvard School of Public Health and was an Exxon research fellow in the Program on Science, Technology, and Society at the Massachusetts Institute of Technology. She was the program head of the Committee on Scientific Freedom and Responsibility of the American Association for the Advancement of Science from 1976 to 1986. She has a B.A. in foreign affairs from the University of Cincinnati.

**Dr. Patrick Kelley** joined the Institute of Medicine (IOM) in July 2003 as the Director of the Board on Global Health. He has subsequently also been appointed the Director of the Board on African Science Academy Development. Dr. Kelley has overseen a portfolio of IOM expert consensus studies and convening activities on subjects as wide ranging as the evaluation of the U.S. emergency plan for international AIDS relief, the role of border quarantine programs for migrants in the 21st century, sustainable surveillance for zoonotic infections, and the programmatic approach to cancer in low- and middle- income countries. He also directs a unique capacity building effort, the African Science Academy Development Initiative, which over ten 10 years aims to strengthen the capacity of African academies to advise their governments on scientific matters. Prior to coming to the National Academies Dr. Kelley served in the U.S. Army for more than 23 years as a physician, residency director, epidemiologist, and program manager. In his last Department of Defense (DoD) position, Dr. Kelley founded and directed the DoD Global Emerging Infections Surveillance and Response System (DoD-GEIS). This responsibility entailed managing surveillance and capacity building partnerships with numerous elements of the federal government and with health ministries in more than 45 developing countries. Dr. Kelley is an experienced communicator having lectured in English or Spanish in more than 20 countries and published more than 64 scholarly papers, book chapters, and monographs. Dr. Kelley obtained his M.D. from the University of Virginia and his Dr.P.H. in epidemiology from the Johns Hopkins School of Hygiene and Public Health.

# Appendix C

# Public Committee Meeting Agendas

Public Information Gathering Session
November 23, 2009
Washington, DC

10:30am       **Opening Remarks**
*Robert Black,* Committee Chair

10:30am–11:15am       **Address from the Office of the Global AIDS Coordinator**
*Michele Moloney-Kitts,* Assistant Coordinator, Office of the Global AIDS
Coordinator, U.S. Department of State

11:15am–12:30pm       **Discussion with Congressional Staff**
*Shellie Bressler*, Senior Professional Staff, Senate Committee on Foreign Relations

*Pearl-Alice Marsh*, Senior Majority Staff, House Committee on Foreign Affairs

12:30pm–3:00pm       **Closed Session**

3:00pm–4:00pm       **Discussion with the U.S. Government Accountability Office**
*David Gootnick,* Director of International Affairs & Trade Unit, U.S.
Government Accountability Office

4:00pm       **Adjournment**
*Bob Black,* Committee Chair

Public Information Gathering Session
January 6–7, 2010
Washington, DC

*Wednesday, January 6, 2010*

6:15pm–8:15pm   **Committee Dinner**
*Sheila Tlou*, Professor of Nursing, University of Botswana, and Former Minister of Health, Republic of Botswana

*Thursday, January 7, 2010*

8:00am            **Arrival and Check-in**

8:30am–8:45am   **Welcoming Remarks**
*Robert Black,* Committee Chair

8:45am–9:15am   **Address from Ambassador Eric Goosby**
*Eric Goosby,* U.S. Global AIDS Coordinator, Office of the U.S. Global AIDS Coordinator

### SESSION 1: OFFICE OF THE GLOBAL AIDS COORDINATOR STRATEGIC INFORMATION PANEL

9:15am–10:45am   **Overview of OGAC Strategic Information Plan**
*Paul Bouey*, Director of Strategic Information, Office of the Global AIDS Coordinator

**Next Generation Indicators**
*Michelle Lee*, Strategic Information Officer, Office of the Global AIDS Coordinator

**Public Health Evaluations**
*Dianna Edgil*, Strategic Information Officer, Office of the Global AIDS Coordinator

**Prevention Evaluation**
*Caroline Ryan*, Director of Program Services and Chief Technical Officer, Office of the Global AIDS Coordinator

**Q&A and Discussion**

10:45am–11:00am  **Break**

## SESSION 2: U.S. GOVERNMENT AGENCY IMPLEMENTERS PANEL
## DATA COLLECTION, OUTCOME/IMPACT EVALUATION, AND APPLICATION FOR PROGRAMMATIC AND POLICY DECISIONS

11:00am–12:00pm    *William Levine*, Associate Director for Science and Acting Chief, Epidemiology and Strategic Information Branch, U.S. Centers for Disease Control and Prevention

*John Novak*, Senior M&E Advisor to the Office of HIV/AIDS, United States Agency for International Development

**Q&A and Discussion**

12:00pm–1:00pm    **Lunch**

## SESSION 3: IMPLEMENTER PERSPECTIVES
## DATA COLLECTION, OUTCOME/IMPACT EVALUATION, AND APPLICATION FOR PROGRAMMATIC AND POLICY DECISIONS

1:00pm–3:15pm    *Mary Fanning*, Health Attaché and the PEPFAR Coordinator, U.S. Embassy in South Africa
*Phyllis Kanki*, Professor of Immunology and Infectious Diseases, Harvard University
*Carolyn Bolton*, Deputy Medical Director, Centers for Infectious Disease Research, Zambia
*Mary Owens*, Executive Director of The Children of God Relief Institute Nyumbani, Kenya
*Sheila Dinotshe Tlou*, Professor of Nursing, University of Botswana, and Former Minister of Health, Republic of Botswana

**Q&A and Discussion**

3:15pm–3:30pm    **Break**

## SESSION 4: BEST PRACTICES AND LESSONS LEARNED FROM LARGE-SCALE PROGRAM EVALUATION

3:30pm–6:00pm    **IOM PEPFAR Design Considerations Workshop**
*Ruth Levine*, Vice President for Programs and Operations, Center for Global Development

**Global Fund Evaluation**
*Martin Vaessen*, Director, Demographic and Health Research Division, ICF Macro

**Evaluation of Health Systems in Africa**
*Lola Dare*, Executive Secretary, African Council for Sustainable Health Development

**Q&A and Discussion**

6:00pm    **Closing Remarks and Adjournment of Public Session**
*Robert Black*, Committee Chair

# Appendix D

# Glossary

|  | | Source |
|---|---|---|
| **Accountability** | Responsibility for the use of resources and the decisions made, as well as the obligation to demonstrate that work has been done in compliance with agreed-upon rules and standards and to report fairly and accurately on performance results vis-à-vis mandated roles and/or plans. | (UNAIDS MERG, 2010, p. 2) |
| **Activities** | Actions taken or work performed through which inputs such as funds, technical assistance, and other types of resources are mobilized to produce specific outputs. | (UNAIDS MERG, 2010, p. 2) |
| **Affordability** | The extent to which countries or people can bear the cost of programs or services. | Adapted from (Merriam-Webster, 2010) |
| **Attribution** | The ascription of a causal link between observed changes and a specific intervention. | (UNAIDS MERG, 2010, p. 2) |
| **Benchmarking** | A systematic process for evaluating the products, services and work processes of organizations that are recognized as representing best practices for the purpose of organizational improvement. | Adapted from (Spendolini, 1992, p. 2 ) |
| **Case study** | A methodological approach that describes a situation, individual, or the like and that typically incorporates data-gathering activities (e.g., interviews, observations, questionnaires) at selected sites or programs/projects. Case studies are characterized by purposive selection of sites or small samples; the | (UNAIDS MERG, 2010, p. 2) |

expectation of generalizability is less than that in many other forms of research. The findings are used to report to stakeholders, make recommendations for program/project improvement, and share lessons learned.

| | | |
|---|---|---|
| **Causal Chain** | A series of statements that link the causes of a problem with its effects (i.e., a causal chain maps the relations between inputs, activities, outputs, outcomes and impact). | (Belausteguigoitia, 2004, p. 2) |
| **CD4 Count** | When HIV actively multiplies, it infects and kills CD4 T cells, a specific type of white blood cell, that are the immune system's key infection fighters. The effects of HIV are measured by the decline in the number of CD4 cells. The CD4 count is the number of CD4 cells in the blood and reflects the state of the immune system. The normal count in a healthy adult is between 600 and 1,200 cells/mm$^3$. | (CDC, 2008, p. 13) |
| **Coordination & Harmonization** | The extent to which donors implement, where feasible, common arrangements at country level for planning, funding (e.g., joint financial arrangements), disbursement, monitoring, evaluating and reporting to government on donor activities and aid flows." | (High-level Forum, 2005, p. 6) |
| **Correlational analysis** | A summary measure of linear association between two quantitative variables. The correlation coefficient takes the value-1 for perfectly negatively correlated data. For perfectly positively correlated data it takes the value unity. The nearer to zero is the correlation coefficient, the less linear the association there is between the two variables. | (Woodward, 2005, p. 456–457) |
| **Cost-effectiveness/ Efficiency** | A measure of how economically resources/inputs (funds, expertise, time, etc.) are converted to results. | (DAC Network on Development Evaluation, 2002, p. 21) |
| **Country Capacity** | The ability of government, the private sector, and civil society to "plan, manage, implement, and account for results of policies and programs." | Partially adapted from (High-level Forum, 2005, p. 5) |

| **Country Ownership** | A situation in which "partner countries exercise effective leadership over their development policies and strategies, and coordinate development actions." Partner countries expect donors to respect country priorities and to invest in country human resources and institutions with the goal of improving or maximizing the use of the country's systems to deliver aid for more rapid effectiveness with developmental aid "[…] to achieve their own economic, social, and environmental goals." As a part of country ownership, partner countries will be more transparent and accountable to donors, their governing bodies, and their citizens by translating their actions into positive impacts on the lives of their citizens and populations. | Partially adapted from (High-level Forum, 2005, p. 3; Accra Agenda for Action, 2008) |
|---|---|---|
| **Coverage** | The extent to which a program/intervention is being implemented in the right places (geographic coverage) and is reaching its intended target population (individual coverage). | (UNAIDS MERG, 2010, p. 2) |
| **Document review** | An intensive literature search, review and synthesis of all relevant documents concerning the program being evaluated. In the case of HIV programs, documents to be considered may typically include national epidemiological reports, official government or other state-level public health and human rights policy reports, non-governmental organization reports, and any other academic or scientific papers related. Findings are usually integrated into the overall findings of the study and/or used to help design a main project. | (Association of Qualitative Research, 2010a; Operario, 2008, p. 13) |
| **Effectiveness** | The extent to which a program/intervention has achieved its objectives under normal conditions in a real-life setting. | (UNAIDS MERG, 2010, p. 2) |
| **Effects** | Results or changes from the program such as changes in knowledge, awareness, skills, attitudes, opinions, aspirations, motivation, behavior, practice, decision making, policies, social action, condition, or status. Effects may be intended and/or unintended: positive and negative. Effects fall along a continuum from proximal (immediate; initial; short-term) to distal effects (ultimate; long-term), often synonymous with impact. | (Taylor-Powell and Henert, 2008) |

| | | |
|---|---|---|
| **Efficacy** | The extent to which an intervention produces the expected results under ideal conditions in a controlled environment. | (UNAIDS MERG, 2010, p. 3) |
| **Efficiency** | A measure of how, economically, inputs (resources such as funds, expertise, time) are converted into results. | (UNAIDS MERG, 2010, p. 3) |
| **Epidemiology** | The study of the magnitude, distribution and determinants of health-related conditions in specific populations, and the application of the results to control health problems. | (UNAIDS MERG, 2010, p. 3) |
| **Evaluation** | The rigorous, scientifically-based collection of information about program/intervention activities, characteristics, and outcomes that determine the merit or worth of the program/intervention. Evaluation studies provide credible information for use in improving programs/interventions, identifying lessons learned, and informing decisions about future resource allocation. | (UNAIDS MERG, 2010, p. 3) |
| **Facility Survey** | A survey of a representative sample of facilities that generally aims to assess the readiness of all elements required to provide services and other aspects of quality of care (e.g., basic infrastructure, drugs, equipment, test kits, client registers, and trained staff). The units of observation are facilities of various types and levels in the same health system. The content of the survey may vary but typically includes a facility inventory and, sometimes, health worker interviews, client exit interviews, and client-provider observations. | (UNAIDS MERG, 2010, p. 3) |
| **Field Work** | The stage of a research project in which data is collected, whether in the form of interviews, group discussions, observations, or materials for cultural analysis. | (Association of Qualitative Research, 2010b) |
| **Focus Group** | Qualitative methodology used to obtain information about the feelings, opinions, perceptions, insights, beliefs, misconceptions, attitudes and receptivity of a group of people concerning an idea or an issue. They include only 8–12 participants relatively homogeneous though unfamiliar to each other. They share in a guided discussion which is informal and last approximately 2 hours. | (McKenzie, 2005, p. 76) |

| | | |
|---|---|---|
| **Generalizability** | The extent to which findings can be assumed to be true for the entire target population, not just the sample of the population under study.<br>Note: To ensure generalizability, the sampling procedure and the data collected need to meet certain methodological standards. | (UNAIDS MERG, 2010, p. 3) |
| **Geographic Information System (GIS)** | A computer mapping and analysis technology consisting of hardware, software, and data allowing large quantities of information to be viewed and analyzed in a geographic context. It has nearly all of the features of a database management system, with a major enhancement. Every item of information in a GIS is tied to a geographic location. | (O'Carroll, 2003, p. 432) |
| **Health Workforce Strengthening** | "Health workers are all people engaged in actions whose primary intent is to protect and improve health. A country's health workforce consists broadly of health service providers and health management and support workers. This includes private as well as public sector health workers; unpaid and paid workers; lay and professional cadres. Countries have enormous variation in the level, skill and gender-mix in their health workforce. Overall, there is a strong positive correlation between health workforce density and service coverage and health outcomes." Strengthening "involves the improvement in a range of capacities including training, supervision and job satisfaction." | (WHO, 2007, p. 16; IOM, 2008, p. 2) |
| **Health Information Systems** | A data system, usually computerized, that routinely collects and reports information about the delivery and cost of health services, and patient demographics and health status. | (UNAIDS MERG, 2010, p. 3) |
| **Health System** | All organizations, people and actions whose primary intent is to promote, restore or maintain health. WHO divided health systems into six operational "building blocks" action framework: services, workforce, information, commodities and technologies, financing, and leadership and governance. | Partially adapted from (WHO, 2007, pp. v & 2) |
| **HIV-Free Infant Survival** | Proportion of children that are alive and free of HIV-infection, which can be measured at 18 months of age. The denominator of this outcome measure consists of the number of children born within the past two years, estimated through the survey component of the | Adapted from (Stringer et al., 2008) |

Demographic and Health Survey. The numerator is based on the same figure, minus the number of children found to be HIV-infected [determined via HIV antibody and deoxyribonucleic acid polymerase chain reaction testing] and the number of children reported to have died (derived via survey methodology).

| | | |
|---|---|---|
| **Impact** | The long-term, cumulative effect of programs/interventions over time on what they ultimately aim to change, such as a change in HIV infection, AIDS-related morbidity and mortality. Note: Impacts at a population-level are rarely attributable to a single program/intervention, but a specific program/intervention may, together with other programs/interventions, contribute to impacts on a population. | (UNAIDS MERG, 2010, p. 3) |
| **Impact Evaluation** | A type of evaluation that assesses the rise and fall of impacts, such as disease prevalence and incidence, as a function of HIV programs/interventions. Impacts on a population seldom can be attributed to a single program/intervention; therefore, an evaluation of impacts on a population generally entails a rigorous design that assesses the combined effects of a number of programs/interventions for at-risk populations. | (UNAIDS MERG, 2010, p. 3) |
| **Incidence** | The number of new cases of a disease that occur in a specified population during a specified time period. | (UNAIDS MERG, 2010, p. 4) |
| **Indicator** | A quantitative or qualitative variable that provides a valid and reliable way to measure achievement, assess performance, or reflect changes connected to an intervention. Note: Single indicators are limited in their utility for understanding program effects (i.e., what is working or is not working, and why?). Indicator data should be collected and interpreted as part of a set of indicators. Indicator sets alone cannot determine the effectiveness of a program or collection of programs; for this, good evaluation designs are necessary. | (UNAIDS MERG, 2010, p. 4) |
| **Inputs** | The financial, human, and material resources used in a program/intervention. | (UNAIDS MERG, 2010, p. 4) |

| | | |
|---|---|---|
| **Intervention** | A specific activity or set of activities intended to bring about change in some aspect(s) of the status of the target population (e.g., HIV risk reduction, improving the quality of service delivery). | (UNAIDS MERG, 2010, p. 4) |
| **Logic Framework** | Management tool used to improve the design of interventions. It involves identifying strategic elements (inputs, outputs, activities, outcomes, impact) and their causal relationships, indicators, and the assumptions of risks that may influence success and failure. It thus facilitates planning, execution, and monitoring and evaluation of an intervention. | (UNAIDS MERG, 2010, p. 4) |
| **M&E (Monitoring and Evaluation) Strategy** | A multi-year implementation strategy for the collection, analysis and use of data needed for program/project management and accountability purposes. The plan describes the data needs linked to a specific program/project; the M&E activities that need to be undertaken to satisfy the data needs and the specific data collection procedures and tools; the standardized indicators that need to be collected for routine monitoring and regular reporting; the components of the M&E system that need to be implemented and the roles and responsibilities of different organizations/individuals in their implementation; how data will used for program/project management and accountability purposes. The plan indicates resource requirement estimates and outlines a strategy for resource mobilization. Note: A national HIV M&E plan is a multi-sectoral, 3–5 year implementation strategy which is developed and regularly updated with the participation of a wide variety of stakeholders from national, sub-national, and service delivery levels. | (UNAIDS MERG, 2010, p. 4) |
| **Modeling** | Mathematical analysis that describes the association between exposure, outcome and confounders. Numerous models have been developed and their use depends on a certain set of assumptions. It is generally use when it is necessary to control for many confounding variables. | (Woodward, 2005, p. 427) |
| **Monitoring** | Routine tracking and reporting of priority information about a program/project, its inputs and intended outputs, outcomes and impacts. | (UNAIDS MERG, 2010, p. 4) |

| | | |
|---|---|---|
| **Operational Research** | For service delivery programs, the "systematic and objective assessment of the availability, accessibility, quality, and/or sustainability of services designed to improve service delivery. It assesses only factors that are under the control of program/project managers, such as improving the quality of services, increasing training and supervision of staff members, and adding new service components." | (Adapted from UNAIDS MERG, 2010, p. 5) |
| **Opportunistic Infection** | Protozoan, bacterial, fungal, and viral infections that are more frequent or more severe because of immunosuppression in people with HIV infection or AIDS. When the CD4 count of an adult falls below 200 cells/mm$^3$, the risk of opportunistic infection is high. | (Adapted from CDC, 2008, pp. 13–14) |
| **Outcome** | Short-term and medium-term effect of an intervention's outputs, such as change in knowledge, attitudes, beliefs, behaviours. | (UNAIDS MERG, 2010, p. 5) |
| **Outputs** | The results of program/intervention activities; the direct products or deliverables of program/intervention activities, such as the number of HIV counseling sessions completed, the number of people served, the number of condoms distributed. | (UNAIDS MERG, 2010, p. 5) |
| **Pilot Test** | A set of procedures used by planners/evaluators to try out various processes during program development on a small group of subjects prior to actual implementation. | (McKenzie, 2005, p. 123) |
| **Population-based Survey** | A type of survey which is statistically representative of the target population, such as the AIDS Indicator Survey and the Demographic and Health Survey. | (UNAIDS MERG, 2010, p. 5) |
| **Prevalence** | The total number of persons living with a specific disease or condition at a given time. | (UNAIDS MERG, 2010, p. 5) |
| **Program** | An overarching national or sub-national response to a disease. A program generally includes a set of interventions marshaled to attain specific global, regional, country, or sub-national objectives; involves multiple activities that may cut across sectors, themes and/or geographic areas. | (UNAIDS MERG, 2010, p. 5) |

| | | |
|---|---|---|
| **Program Evaluation** | "A study that intends to control a health problem or improve a public health program or service. The intended benefits of the program are primarily or exclusively for the study participants or the study participants' community (i.e., the population from which the study participants were sampled); data collected are needed to assess and/or improve the program or service, and/or the health of the study participants or the study participants' community. Knowledge that is generated does not typically extend beyond the population or program from which data are collected." Also referred to as summative evaluation. | (UNAIDS MERG, 2010, p. 6) |
| **Qualitative Data** | Data collected using qualitative methods, such as in-depth, open-ended interviews, direct observation, and analysis of written documents. Qualitative data can provide an understanding of social situations and interactions, as well as people's values, perceptions, motivations, and reactions. Qualitative data are generally expressed in narrative form, pictures or objects (i.e., not numerically). When using mixed methods, "findings may be presented either alone or in combination with quantitative data." There are many different theoretical perspectives for qualitative inquiry, but they all attempt to describe or explain phenomena. | (Adapted from UNAIDS MERG, 2010, p. 6; Patton, 2002, p. 4, 5) |
| **Qualitative Interview Methods** | Include individual and group approaches to data collection. They feature in-depth and extended discussions guided by an interviewer. They vary in the degree of structure involved. On one end of the continuum are semi-structured interviews using predefined questions that allow open-ended responses. Open-ended interviews are less structured and use a list of discussion topics to cover in each interview. Least structured are the informal interviews. | (Sankar et al., 2006, p.s55) |
| **Quantitative Data** | Data collected using quantitative methods, such as surveys. Quantitative data are measured on a numerical scale, can be analyzed using statistical methods, and can be displayed using tables, charts, histograms and graphs. The aim of a quantitative study is to classify features, count them, and construct statistical models in an attempt to explain what is observed. | (UNAIDS MERG, 2010, p. 6) |

| | | |
|---|---|---|
| **Quasi-Experimental Study** | Study in which comparisons are made between nonequivalent groups that are not randomly assigned to intervention and control groups. | Epidemiology GORDIS |
| **Randomized Controlled Trial** | Study where subjects are allocated to intervention and control groups according to some chance mechanism. | (Woodward, 2005, p. 343) |
| **Research** | A study which intends to generate or contribute to generalizable knowledge to improve public health practice, i.e., the study intends to generate new information that has relevance beyond the population or program from which data are collected. Research typically attempts to make statements about how the different variables under study, in controlled circumstances, affect one another at a given point in time. | (UNAIDS MERG, 2010, p. 6) |
| **Results** | The outputs, outcomes, or impacts (intended or unintended, positive and/or negative) of an intervention. | (UNAIDS MERG, 2010, p. 6) |
| **Stakeholder** | A person, group, or entity that has a direct or indirect role and interest in the goals or objectives and implementation of a program/intervention and/or its evaluation. | (UNAIDS MERG, 2010, p. 7) |
| **Summative Evaluation** | A type of evaluation conducted at the end of an intervention (or a phase of that intervention) to determine the extent to which anticipated outcomes were produced. It is designed to provide information about the merit or worth of the intervention. | (UNAIDS MERG, 2010, p. 7) |
| **Surveillance** | The ongoing, systematic collection, analysis, interpretation, and dissemination of data regarding a specific disease or behavior for use in public health action to reduce morbidity and mortality and to improve health. These kinds of surveillance data can help predict future trends and target needed prevention and treatment programs. | (Adapted from UNAIDS MERG, 2010, p. 7) |
| **Sustainability** | The continuation of benefits from a development intervention after major development assistance has been completed. | (DAC Network on Development Evaluation, 2002, p. 36) |
| **Systematic Literature** | "A collation of all empirical evidence that fits pre-specified eligibility criteria to answer a specific | (Adapted from Liberati, et al., |

| | | |
|---|---|---|
| **Review** | research question. It uses explicit, systematic methods that are selected with a view to minimizing bias, thus providing reliable findings from which conclusions can be drawn and decisions made. The key characteristics of a systematic review are: (a) a clearly stated set of objectives with an explicit, reproducible methodology; (b) a systematic search that attempts to identify all studies that would meet the eligibility criteria; (c) an assessment of the validity of the findings of the included studies, for example through the assessment of risk of bias; and (d) systematic presentation, and synthesis, of the characteristics and findings of the included studies." These methods can be applied to various types of literature for research. | 2009, p. 2) |
| **Trend Analysis** | Statistical techniques used for analyzing data over time. The primary step is to plot the observed numbers or rates of interest by study period, followed by further inspection of the data which provides the basis for subsequent analysis including data transformation and smoothing, and more complex statistical procedures (regression analysis, time series analysis). | Adapted from (Rosenberg, 1997) |
| **Triangulation** | The analysis of data from three or more sources obtained by different methods. Findings can be corroborated, and the weakness or bias of any of the methods or data sources can be compensated for by the strengths of another, thereby increasing the validity and reliability of the results. Data triangulation, investigator triangulation, and theory triangulation are three other types of this analytic technique. While ideal, the technique can be expensive—"a study's limited budget and time will affect the amount of triangulation that is practical." | (Adapted from UNAIDS MERG, 2010, p. 7, Patton, 2002, p. 247.) |
| **Validity** | The extent to which a measurement or test accurately measures what is intended to be measured. | (UNAIDS MERG, 2010, p. 7) |

## GLOSSARY REFERENCES

Association of Qualitative Research. 2010a. *"Desk Research."*
    http://www.aqr.org.uk/glossary/?term=deskresearch (accessed June 7, 2010).
Association of Qualitative Research. 2010b. *"Fieldwork."*
    http://www.aqr.org.uk/glossary/?term=fieldwork (accessed June 7, 2010).
Belausteguigoitia JC. 2004. Causal chain analysis and root causes: the GIWA approach. *Ambio* 33(1–2):7–12.

CDC (Centers for Disease Control and Prevention). 2008. *PMTCT training programme trainer manual. Module 1: Introduction to HIV/AIDS.* Washington, DC: CDC.

DAC (Development Assistance Committee) Network on Development Evaluation. 2002. *Glossary of key terms in evaluation and results based management, evaluation and aid effectiveness.* Paris: Organisation for Economic Co-operation and Development.

High-Level Forum. 2005. *Paris declaration on aid effectiveness: Ownership, harmonization, alignment, results, and mutual accountability,* Paris, France, February 28-March 2.

High-Level Forum. 2008. *Accra agenda for action,* Third High-Level Forum on Aid Effectiveness, Accra, Ghana, September 2–4.

IOM (Institute of Medicine). 2008. *Design considerations for evaluating the impact of PEPFAR.* Washington, DC: The National Academies Press.

Liberati, A., D. G. Altman, J. Tetzlaff, C. Mulrow, P. C. Gotzsche, J. P. Ioannidis, M. Clarke, P. J. Devereaux, J. Kleijnen, and D. Moher. 2009. The PRISMA statement for reporting systematic reviews and meta-analyses of studies that evaluate health care interventions: Explanation and elaboration. *PLoS Med* 6(7):e1000100.

MacKenzie, J. F., B. L. Neiger, J. L. and Smeltzer. 2005. *Planning, implementing & evaluating health promotion programs—A primer.* 4ed. San Francisco, CA: Benjamin Cummings.

Merriam-Webster. 2010. *"Affordability."* http://mw2.merriam-webster.com/dictionary/affordability. (accessed June 16, 2010).

O'Carroll, W. Yasnoff, and M. E. Ward. 2003. *Public health informatics and information systems.* New York: Springer-Verlag.

Operario, D. 2008. *Guideline for a qualitative research methodology to assess the social impacts of HIV and identify priorities for advocacy action.* Bratislava, Slovakia: United Nations Development Programme Bratislava Regional Centre.

Patton, M. Q. 2002. *Qualitative research & evaluation methods,* 3rd edition. Thousand Oaks, CA: Sage Publications, Inc.

Rosenberg, D. 1997. *Trend analysis and interpretation: Key concepts and methods for maternal and child health professionals.* Rockville, MD: Health Resources and Services Administration.

Sankar, A., C. Golin, J. M. Simoni, M. Luborsky, and C. Pearson. 2006. How qualitative methods contribute to understanding combination antiretroviral therapy adherence. *J Acquir Immune Defic Syndr* 43(Suppl 1):S54–S68.

Spendolini, J. M. 1992. *The benchmarking book.* New York: American Management Association.

Stringer, E. M., B. H. Chi, N. Chintu, T. L. Creek, D. K. Ekouevi, D. Coetzee, P. Tih, A. Boulle, F. Dabis, N. Shaffer, C. M. Wilfert, and J. S. Stringer. 2008. Monitoring effectiveness of programmes to prevent mother-to-child HIV transmission in lower-income countries. *Bull World Health Organ* 86(1):57–62.

Taylor-Powell, E. and E. Henert. 2008. *Developing a logic model: Teaching and training guide.* Madison, WI: University of Wisconsin.

UNAIDS MERG (United Nations Joint Programme on HIV/AIDS Monitoring and Evaluation Reference Group). 2010. *Glossary: monitoring and evaluation terms.* Geneva, Switzerland: UNAIDS.

WHO (World Health Organization). 2007. *Everybody's business: Strengthening health systems to improve health outcomes-WHO's framework for action.* Geneva, Switzerland: WHO.

Woodward, M. 2005. *Epidemiology—Study design and data analysis.* 2nd ed. Boca Raton, FL: Chapman & Hall/CRC Press.

# Appendix E

# Sample PEPFAR Country Timelines

176

# Botswana

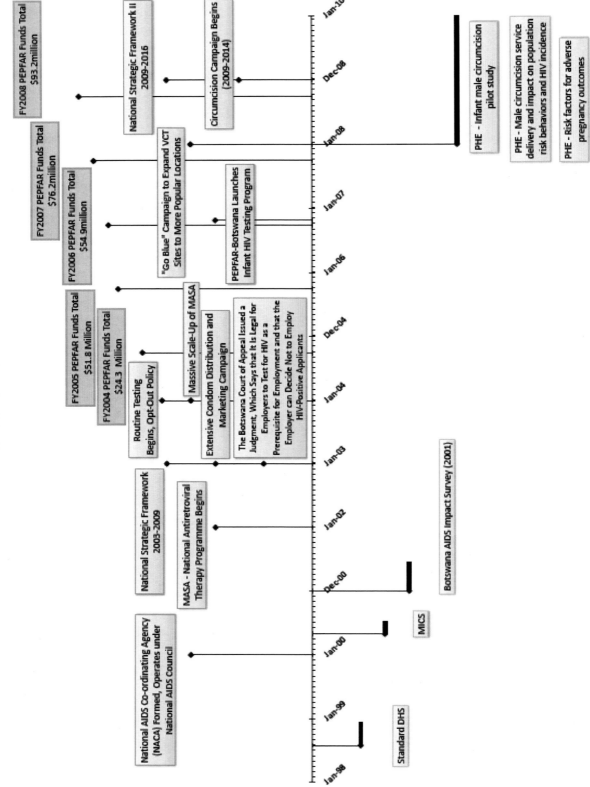

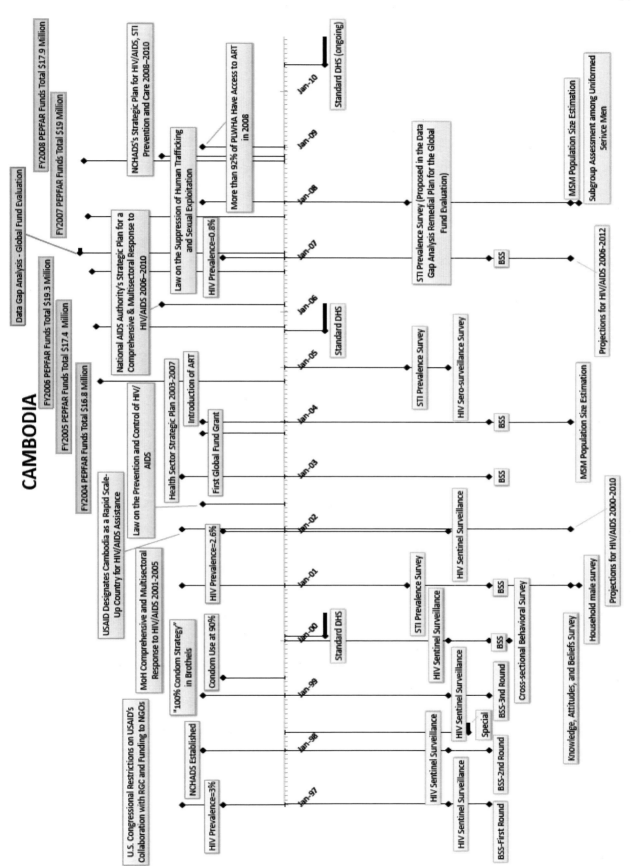

178

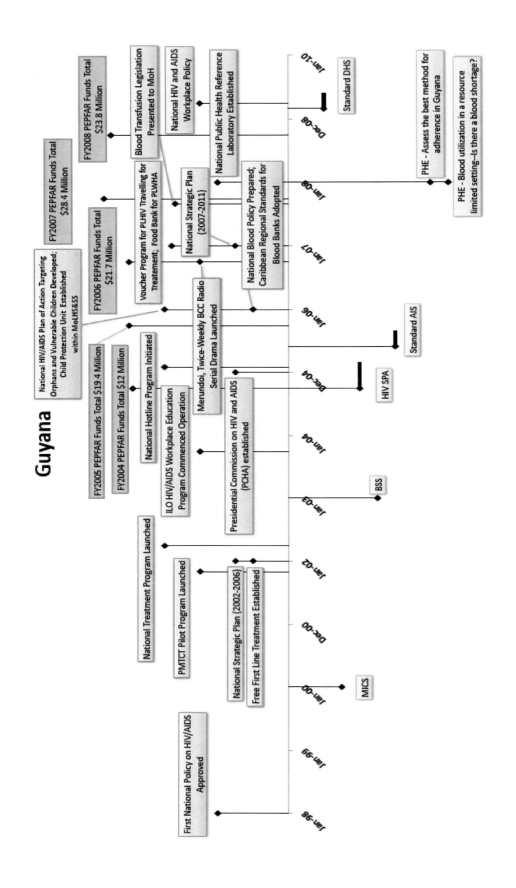

Guyana

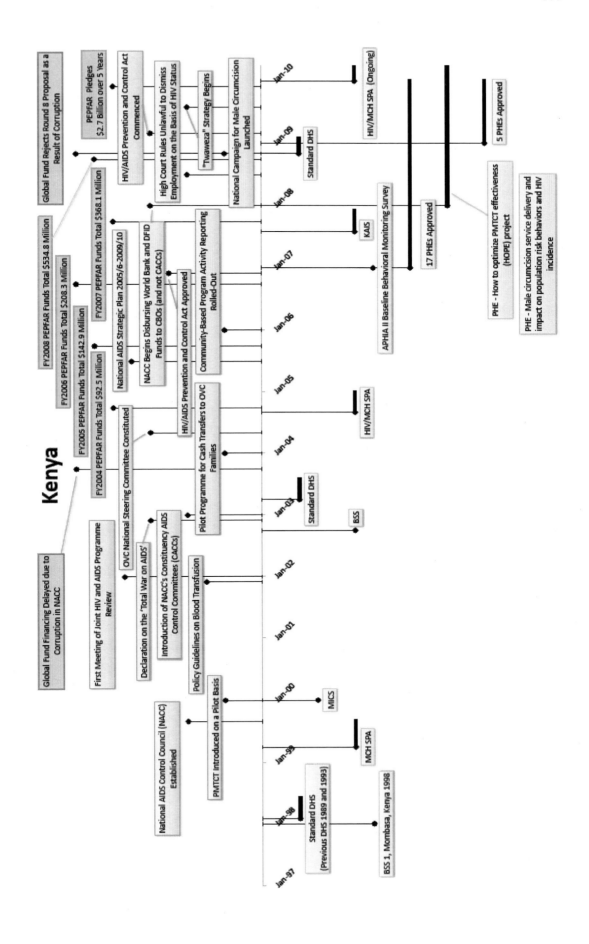

Kenya

Global Fund Financing Delayed due to Corruption in NACC

First Meeting of Joint HIV and AIDS Programme Review

OVC National Steering Committee Constituted

Declaration on the "Total War on AIDS"

Introduction of NACC's Constituency AIDS Control Committees (CACCs)

Policy Guidelines on Blood Transfusion

National AIDS Control Council (NACC) Established

PMTCT Introduced on a Pilot Basis

Global Fund Rejects Round 8 Proposal as a Result of Corruption

PEPFAR Pledges $2.7 Billion over 5 Years

HIV/AIDS Prevention and Control Act Commenced

High Court Rules Unlawful to Dismiss Employment on the Basis of HIV Status

"Twaweza" Strategy Begins

National Campaign for Male Circumcision Launched

FY2008 PEPFAR Funds Total $534.8 Million

FY2006 PEPFAR Funds Total $208.3 Million

FY2007 PEPFAR Funds Total $368.1 Million

National AIDS Strategic Plan 2005/6-2009/10

NACC Begins Disbursing World Bank and DFID Funds to CBOs (and not CACCs)

Community-Based Program Activity Reporting Rolled-Out

FY2005 PEPFAR Funds Total $142.9 Million

FY2004 PEPFAR Funds Total $92.5 Million

HIV/AIDS Prevention and Control Act Approved

HIV/AIDS Prevention and Control Act Transfers to OVC

Pilot Programme for Cash Transfers to OVC Families

Standard DHS (Previous DHS 1989 and 1993)

BSS 1, Mombasa, Kenya 1998

MCH SPA

MICS

Standard DHS

BSS

HIV/MCH SPA

HIV/MCH SPA

Standard DHS

KAIS

APHIA II Baseline Behavioral Monitoring Survey

17 PHEs Approved

5 PHEs Approved

HIV/MCH SPA (Ongoing)

PHE - How to optimize PMTCT effectiveness (HOPE) project

PHE - Male circumcision service delivery and impact on population risk behaviors and HIV incidence

Jan-97  Jan-98  Jan-99  Jan-00  Jan-01  Jan-02  Jan-03  Jan-04  Jan-05  Jan-06  Jan-07  Jan-08  Jan-09  Jan-10

## Country Timelines

*List of Abbreviations in the Country Timelines*

**Botswana** DHS = Demographic and Health Survey; FY = fiscal year; MICS = Multiple Indicator Cluster Survey; PHE = public health evaluation; VCT = voluntary counseling and testing.

**Cambodia** ART = antiretroviral therapy; BSS = Behavioral Health Survey; DHS = Demographic and Health Survey; FY = fiscal year; MoH = Ministry of Health; MSM = men who have sex with men; NCHADS = National Center for HIV/AIDS, Dermatology and STD; NGO = non-governmental organization; PLWHA = people living with HIV/AIDS; RGC = Royal Government of Cambodia; STI = sexually transmitted infection; USAID = United States Agency for International Development.

**Guyana** AIS = AIDS Indicator Survey; BCC = behavior change communication; BSS = Behavioral Health Survey; DHS = Demographic and Health Survey; FY = fiscal year; ILO = International Labor Organization; MICS = Multiple Indicator Cluster Survey; MoH = Ministry of Health; MoLHS&SS = Ministry of Labor, Human Services, and Social Security; PHE = public health evaluation; PLHIV = people living with HIV/AIDS; PMTCT = prevention of mother-to-child-transmission; SPA = Service Provision Assessment Survey.

**Kenya** APHIA = AIDS, Population and Health Integrated Assistance II project; BSS = Behavioral Health Survey; CBO = community-based organization; DFID = UK Department for International Development; DHS = Demographic and Health Survey; FY = fiscal year; MCH SPA = Maternal and Child Health Service Provision Assessment Survey; KAIS = Kenya AIDS Indicator Survey; MICS = Multiple Indicator Cluster Survey; PHE = public health evaluation; PMTCT = prevention of mother-to-child transmission; OVC = orphans and vulnerable children.

*Research Process and Methodology*

An initial broad scan was conducted between December 2009 and January 2010 to retrieve information for the four countries presented in this Appendix. The countries selected for the initial research are part of the 31 COP countries[1] for FY2009 (i.e., countries that submitted a country operational plan (COP) to PEPFAR in fiscal year 2009). At the beginning of this activity, the COP process for FY2010 was ongoing. The information collected for each country extends, at least, for the past 12 years. The information was drawn from published and gray literature primarily from OGAC and U.S. agencies including PEPFAR implementing agencies and partners (e.g., USAID and Family Health International), in-country sources such as the 2008 UNGASS reports, and other global stakeholders reports (e.g., Global Fund and UNAIDS). Additionally, global health or health policy media outlets were used as a source of information on current events related to the HIV/AIDS epidemic in the different countries. The main types of information gathered through the document identification and screening process to build the country timelines for Botswana, Cambodia, Guyana, and Kenya included PEPFAR activities and/or investment, Global Fund HIV/AIDS-related activities and investments, country-level

---

[1] In FY2009, the Caribbean region submitted a COP but for purposes of the research and development of the country timelines, it was not considered a country.

policy information in connection with the national HIV/AIDS response, as well as information about recent data collection activities such as population-based surveys and other HIV/AIDS-related surveillance either already completed or proposed.

*Limitations*

The format and design of the timeline limits the number of activities or events represented in each of the country timelines. Therefore, the country events included after the completion of the research were prioritized, and only a subset of the country events was included in the country timeline figure (snapshot). Additionally, these country snapshots only presents a number of events related to the national HIV/AIDS response and are not intended to be comprehensive. The information for these timelines was available in a number of different locations (documents, websites, and databases), and thus the research and initial scan of information was limited to the documents and databases listed below.

*Documents and Databases Reviewed*

AVERT. 2010. *HIV & AIDS in Botswana*. Last updated May 17, 2010.
    http://www.avert.org/aids-botswana.htm (accessed June 9, 2010).
AVERT. 2010. *Asia AIDS timeline*. Last updated March 12, 2010. http://www.avert.org/asia-
    aids-timeline.htm (accessed June 11, 2010).
Botswana Ministry of State President, and National AIDS Coordinating Agency. 2008. *Progress*
    *report of the national response to the UNGASS Declaration of Commitment on    HIV/AIDS*.
    http://data.unaids.org/pub/Report/2008/botswana_2008_country_progress_report_en.pdf
    (accessed June 11, 2010).
Canadian HIV/AIDS Legal Network. http://www.aidslaw.ca/EN/index.htm (accessed June 9,      2010).
Christopher, S., and M. Kunthear. 2009. Cambodian report damns law for confusing trafficking
    with sex work. *The Phnom Penh Post*, June 23.
    http://www.nodo50.org/Laura_Agustin/cambodian-report-damns-trafficking-law-for-mixing-up-
    trafficking-with-sex-work (accessed June 11, 2010).
FHI (Family Health International). *BSS/BBSS studies conducted by Family Health International,*
    *1989–2009*.http://www.fhi.org/en/HIVAIDS/pub/survreports/res_BSS_full_list.htm
    (accessed June 8, 2010).
GFTAM (The Global Fund to Fight AIDS, Tuberculosis, and Malaria). 2010. *Grant*
    *portfolio: Cambodia*. http://portfolio.theglobalfund.org/Country/Index/CAM?lang=en (accessed
    June 11, 2010).
Government of Guyana National HIV/AIDS Programme. 2009. *HIV/AIDS in Guyana (last*
    *updated November 19, 2009)*. http://www.hiv.gov.gy/gp_hiv_gy.php (accessed June 11, 2010).
International AIDS Alliance. *Khmer HIV/AIDS NGO Alliance (KHANA)*.
    http://www.aidsalliance.org/linkingorganisationdetails.aspx?id=5 (accessed June 11, 2010).
IRIN (The Integrated Regional Information Networks). 2008. Kenya: Global Fund rejection
    brings a rethink. PlusNews, October 29. http://www.plusnews.org/report.aspx?ReportID=81188
    (accessed June 11, 2010).
IRIN. 2009. Global: Falling foul of the fund. PlusNews, November 11.
    http://www.plusnews.org/Report.aspx?ReportId=86972 (accessed June 11, 2010).
IRIN. 2009. Kenya: Meeting Muslim leaders halfway on HIV education. PlusNews, December 8.
    http://www.plusnews.org/Report.aspx?ReportId=87367 (accessed June 11, 2010).
IRIN. 2009. Kenya: The million man cut. PlusNews, November 19.
    http://www.plusnews.org/Report.aspx?ReportId=87074 (accessed June 11, 2010).

IRIN. 2009. Kenya: PEPFAR doubles AIDS funding. PlusNews, December 17. http://www.plusnews.org/Report.aspx?ReportId=87468 (accessed June 11, 2010).

KFF (Kaiser Family Foundation). 2006. Botswana launches infant HIV testing program. Kaiser Daily HIV/AIDS Report, October 27. http://dailyreports.kff.org/Daily-Reports/2006/October/27/dr00040699.aspx (accessed June 9, 2010).

KFF. 2009. Global challenges: Botswana health officials announce HIV-prevention project to circumcise 80 percent of eligible men over five years. Kaiser Daily HIV/AIDS Report, May 11. http://www.kaisernetwork.org/daily_reports/rep_index.cfm?hint=1&DR_ID=58395 (accessed June 9, 2010).

KFF. 2009. Drug access: Cambodia reports increase in antiretroviral treatment access. Kaiser Daily HIV/AIDS Report, Jan 28. http://www.kaisernetwork.org/daily_reports/rep_index.cfm?hint=1&DR_ID=56660 (accessed June 11, 2010).

MEASURE DHS (Demographic and Health Surveys). *All surveys by country.* http://www.measuredhs.com/aboutsurveys/search/search_survey_main.cfm?SrvyTp=cou ntry (accessed June 9, 2010).

MEASURE DHS. *HIV/AIDS survey indicators database.* http://www.measuredhs.com/hivdata/ (accessed June 9, 2010).

MLHS & SS (Ministry of Labour, Human Services and Social Services, Guyana). 2009. *HIV/AIDS in the workplace* http://www.hiv.gov.gy/workplace.php (accessed June 11, 2010).

NACC (National AIDS Control Council, Office of the President, Kenya). 2007. *About NACC – History.* http://www.nacc.or.ke/2007/default2.php?active_page_id=117 (updated June 11, 2010).

NACC. 2008. *UNGASS 2008 United Nations General Assembly Special Session on HIV and AIDS: Country report, Kenya. Reporting period: January 2006–December 2007.* Nairobi: NACC. http://data.unaids.org/pub/Report/2008/kenya_2008_country_progress_report_en.pdf (accessed June 11, 2010).

Ndadi, U. 2008. HIV/AIDS and employment law in Botswana. *Botswana Review of Ethics, Law and HIV/AIDS* 2(1).

NCHADS (The National Centre for HIV/AIDS Dermatology and STDs, Cambodia). 2010. *NCHADS: Mission, functions and structure.* http://www.nchads.org/index.php?id=25 (accessed June 11, 2010).

NCHADS. 2001. *Behavioral surveillance survey (BSS) 1997–1999.* Phnom Penh: NCHADS. http://www.nchads.org/Publication/BSS/bss97-99.pdf (accessed June 11, 2010).

PEPFAR (The United States President's Emergency Plan for AIDS Relief). 2010. *Partnership to fight HIV/AIDS in Botswana.* http://www.pepfar.gov/countries/botswana/index.htm (accessed June 9, 2010).

PEPFAR. 2010. *Partnership to fight HIV/AIDS in Cambodia.* http://www.pepfar.gov/countries/cambodia/index.htm (accessed June 11, 2010).

PEPFAR. 2010. *Partnership to fight HIV/AIDS in Guyana.* http://www.pepfar.gov/countries/guyana/index.htm (accessed June 11, 2010).

PEPFAR. 2010. *Partnership to fight HIV/AIDS in Kenya.* http://www.pepfar.gov/countries/kenya/index.htm (accessed June 11, 2010).

Presidential Commission on HIV and AIDS (Republic of Guyana). 2008. *UNGASS country progress report. Reporting period: January 2006–December 2007.* http://data.unaids.org/pub/Report/2008/guyana_2008_country_progress_report_en.pdf (accessed June 11, 2010).

Sou, S., P. Tia, and C. L. Ward. 2004. *Implementing Cambodia's law on the prevention and control of HIV/AIDS.* Abstract presented at the 15th International Conference on AIDS, Bangkok, Thailand, July 11–16. http://gateway.nlm.nih.gov/MeetingAbstracts/ma?f=102280454.html (accessed June 11, 2010).

USAID. 2004. *Cambodia HIV/AIDS Strategic Plan 2002–2005.*
    http://www.usaid.gov/kh/health/documents/USAID_Cambodia_HIV_strategy_2002_200 5.pdf
    (accessed June 11, 2010).
USAID. 2008. *USAID Cambodia: HIV/AIDS health profile.*
    http://www.usaid.gov/our_work/global_health/aids/Countries/asia/cambodia_profile.pdf
    (accessed June 11, 2010).

# Appendix F

# Evaluation Committee Workplan

| Major Activity | 2010 | | | | | | 2011 | | | | | |
|---|---|---|---|---|---|---|---|---|---|---|---|---|
| | Q3 | | | Q4 | | | Q1 | | | Q2 | | |
| Staffing initiated and evaluation committee slate proposed | ■ | ■ | ■ | | | | | | | | | |
| Evaluation committee appointed | ■ | ■ | ■ | ■ | | | | | | | | |
| Meeting #1 planning | ■ | | | | | | | | | | | |
| Committee meeting #1 (Washington, DC) | | | ■ | | | | | | | | | |
| Qualitative methods contractor activity (staff training, committee and country visits analysis: varying intensity in activities) | ■ | ■ | ■ | ■ | ■ | | | | | | | |
| Qualitative methods training for committee and continued review and analyses of data collected during pilot site visits conducted during operational plan period of Summer 2010 | | | ■ | | | | | | | | | |
| Operational Planning Phase—All Activities | ■ | ■ | ■ | | | | | | | | | |
| First country visit (1 of 14) | | | ■ | ■ | | | | | | | | |
| Feedback and data analysis from country visit #1 | | | | ■ | ■ | | | | | | | |
| Committee consultation with global stakeholders | | | | | ■ | | | | | | | |
| Additional staffing (as needed) | | | | | | | ■ | | | | | |
| Committee meeting #2 | | | | | | | ■ | | | | | |
| Country visits (2 of 14) (this is subject to change if concurrent trips are possible) | | | | | | | | ■ | ■ | ■ | ■ | ■ |
| Additional data collection, analysis and consultation with country visits teams, subcontractors, and global/country stakeholders; begin report drafting | | | | | | | ■ | ■ | ■ | ■ | ■ | ■ |
| Committee consultation with global stakeholders | | | | | | | ■ | | | | | |
| Committee meeting #3 | | | | | | | | | | | | |
| Potential committee meeting #4 | | | | | | | | | | | | |
| Continued data collection, syntheses, and mixed-method analyses by committee, staff, and subcontractors | | | | | | | | | | | | |
| Last collection of PEPFAR data for analysis | | | | | | | | | | | | |
| Virtual meeting #5 | | | | | | | | | | | | |
| Committee deliberations and continued report drafting | | | | | | | | | | | | |
| Virtual meeting #6 | | | | | | | | | | | | |
| Enter report review | | | | | | | | | | | | |
| Response to review comments | | | | | | | | | | | | |
| Report sign off | | | | | | | | | | | | |
| Report production | | | | | | | | | | | | |
| Deliver report to sponsor | | | | | | | | | | | | |
| Sponsor and potential Congressional briefings (as requested) | | | | | | | | | | | | |
| Public briefing and report dissemination | | | | | | | | | | | | |

| 2011 | | | | | | 2012 | | | | | | | | | | | |
|------|--|--|--|--|--|------|--|--|--|--|--|--|--|--|--|--|--|
| Q3 | | | Q4 | | | Q1 | | | Q2 | | | Q3 | | | Q4 | | |

# Appendix G

# Sample Data Sources Matrix

**TABLE G-1** Data Sources for PEPFAR Countries 2004–2012

| Countries [N=31] | PEPFAR Indicators (Input/Output/Outcome/Impact) [N=31] | Program Data from Country Operational Plans/Reports [N=31] | OGAC Natural Experiments* [N=?] | Data from Implementing Partners [N=?] |
| --- | --- | --- | --- | --- |
| Angola | | | | |
| Botswana | | | | |
| Cambodia | | | | |
| China | | | | |
| Congo, DR | | | | |
| Côte d'Ivoire | | | | |
| Dominican Republic | | | | |
| Ethiopia | | | | |
| Ghana | | | | |
| Guyana | | | | |
| Haiti | | | | |
| India | | | | |
| Indonesia | | | | |
| Kenya | | | | |
| Lesotho | | | | |
| Malawi | | | | |
| Mozambique | | | | |
| Namibia | | | | |
| Nigeria | | | | |
| Russia | | | | |
| Rwanda | | | | |
| South Africa | | | | |
| Sudan | | | | |
| Swaziland | | | | |
| Tanzania | | | | |
| Thailand | | | | |
| Uganda | | | | |
| Ukraine | | | | |
| Vietnam | | | | |
| Zambia | | | | |
| Zimbabwe | | | | |

NOTE: *Situations where outcome data has been collected systematically by OGAC as program funding became available and after.

OGAC = Office of the U.S. Global AIDS Coordinator, PEPFAR = The President's Emergency Plan for AIDS Relief.

**TABLE G-2** Data Sources for PEPFAR Countries (2004–2012)

| Countries [N=31] | Public Health Evaluations [N=?] | Country Visit Data [N=12–15] | Global Partner Data (e.g., UNGASS/ UNAIDS, Global Fund, World Bank) [N=31] | National Population Surveys (e.g., DHS, MICS) [N=?] | Impact Modeling [N=31] |
|---|---|---|---|---|---|
| Angola | | | | | |
| Botswana | | | | | |
| Cambodia | | | | | |
| China | | | | | |
| Congo, DR | | | | | |
| Côte d'Ivoire | | | | | |
| Dominican Republic | | | | | |
| Ethiopia | | | | | |
| Ghana | | | | | |
| Guyana | | | | | |
| Haiti | | | | | |
| India | | | | | |
| Indonesia | | | | | |
| Kenya | | | | | |
| Lesotho | | | | | |
| Malawi | | | | | |
| Mozambique | | | | | |
| Namibia | | | | | |
| Nigeria | | | | | |
| Russia | | | | | |
| Rwanda | | | | | |
| South Africa | | | | | |
| Sudan | | | | | |
| Swaziland | | | | | |
| Tanzania | | | | | |
| Thailand | | | | | |
| Uganda | | | | | |
| Ukraine | | | | | |
| Vietnam | | | | | |
| Zambia | | | | | |
| Zimbabwe | | | | | |

NOTE: DHS = Demographic and Health Surveys, Global Fund=The Global Fund to Fight AIDS, Tuberculosis and Malaria, MICS = Multiple Indicator Cluster Survey, UNAIDS = Joint United Nations Programme on HIV/AIDS, UNGASS = United Nations General Assembly Special Session.

# Appendix H

# Illustrative Questions for the Evaluation of PEPFAR's Health Systems Strengthening Activities

| WHO HSS Building Block | PEPFAR Inputs | Activities | Outputs | Outcomes | Impacts |
|---|---|---|---|---|---|
| Finance | To what extent has PEPFAR-funded government HIV, non-HIV, and non-health programs? | What specific PEPFAR activities are aimed at reducing the cost, and/or improving the cost-effectiveness or affordability of the health system?<br><br>How is PEPFAR coordinating its financing activities with other donors and partners? | What has been the balance between PEPFAR funding on prevention and treatment?<br><br>What percentage of PEPFAR budgets is channeled through the government versus directly to partners and what share of total financing of government services does this represent? | What has been the trend in the cost per person treated for specific HIV services supported by PEPFAR in the government health system?<br><br>How sustainable is funding for HIV services?<br><br>How have PEPFAR's inputs affected affordability of government health services?<br><br>To what extent do PEPFAR's technical assistance activities contribute to a sound public finance system for health?<br><br>Has PEPFAR improved equity of access to health or AIDS services? Equity in improvements in health? (income and gender) | **What, if any, health improvements can be linked to PEPFAR's activities?** |
| Commodities and Procurement | What infrastructure has been put in place to ensure reliable procurement and supply chain systems?<br><br>How much of this HIV infrastructure (labs, pharmacy, information technology, etc.) is used for non-HIV services (spillover)? | What are the training activities for drug and lab procurement and other supply chain management and pharmacist activities?<br><br>Are PEPFAR supported commodity/procurement activities mainstreamed into public health system services (parallel or integrated) and coordinated with similar multi-donor efforts? | What amount and quality of drugs (and other variable inputs) has PEPFAR financed for use by the public health system?<br><br>To what extent has PEPFAR increased:<br>-access to HIV lab services?<br>-availability of HIV testing (ELISA, CD4, viral loads) in public labs?<br><br>What is the quality of HIV and non-HIV lab services in country (QA certification)? | How have PEPFAR activities affected:<br>-health service forecasting?<br>- procurement and delivery of HIV and non-HIV drugs services (e.g., for tuberculosis, malaria, pain, cancer, cardiovascular disease)?<br>-national essential drug list?<br>-health service ability to run HIV services based on CD4 count testing, viral load testing<br>-functionality of country's supply chain system for high quality, reliable HIV and non-HIV services? | **What, if any, health improvements can be linked to PEPFAR's activities?** |

| | | | | | What, if any, health improvements can be linked to PEPFAR's activities? |
|---|---|---|---|---|---|
| *Information systems* | What has PEPFAR introduced to improve monitoring and evaluation of HIV care systems, HR and health management systems, and decision making? | What activities has PEPFAR undertaken to introduce new data systems or to strengthen existing health information systems that support HIV and non-HIV programs? | What is the functionality of the health information systems supporting HIV and non-HIV programs, and what the number of information officers trained? What new publicly available data and/or research has PEPFAR-funded that could be used by governments to improve the effectiveness of AIDS or health programs? | What is the evidence that the health information and surveillance systems supported by PEPFAR are being used and are functioning better as a result of PEPFAR activities? To what extent has capacity been built and retained to carry on these tasks in the absence of PEPFAR support? To what extent has PEPFAR contributed to a high functioning, single data system for quality-driven health system performance? | What, if any, health improvements can be linked to PEPFAR's activities? |
| *Service delivery* | What resources has PEPFAR added to improve service delivery for HIV and non-HIV services (personnel, buildings, technical assistance, etc.) and to what extent has this support been appropriate for resource-constrained environments? | For HIV and non-HIV care, what activities have PEPFAR undertaken to: -strengthen referral systems and care networks? -use continuous quality improvement methods? -design scalable (rate, cost) and equitable services? -integrate HIV and non-HIV care? | To what extent have PEPFAR's HIV services been decentralized and scaled up in a geographic area? To what extent are leaders of the health system and health care workers using CQI to manage and execute HIV and non-HIV programs? | Are PEPFARs activities linked to effective, efficient, safe, equitable and, patient-centered HIV and non-HIV care? Can PEPFAR HIV and non-HIV programs show improvement in performance and quality of processes and outcomes over time? What is the evidence that PEPFAR's investments in the public health system have improved access to HIV and non-HIV preventive or curative health care? Is there a spillover of improvement to non-health sectors? | What, if any, health improvements can be linked to PEPFAR's activities? |

| | | | | What, if any, health improvements can be linked to PEPFAR's activities? |
|---|---|---|---|---|
| *Leadership and Governance* | What countries have developed and signed partnership frameworks and to what extent have leadership and governance activities been specifically funded? | What activities has PEPFAR supported to specifically improve leadership and governance of: -effective and efficient health protocols? -HIV and non-HIV protocols, policy development and programming? -partnership agreements? -interactions with other bilateral and multilaterals to expand training, financing? | What PEPFAR supported improvements in leadership or governance of the public health sector can be identified, such as: -anti-stigma policies enacted -public and private sector programs accredited for HIV care -updates of national HIV plans and guidelines and concordance with WHO recommendations -integration of HIV into maternal and child health, primary care, hospital or portfolios | What is the evidence that PEPFAR's investments have improved: -health system management and leadership or governance capable of planning and implementing effective, integrated health system interventions for HIV and non-HIV programs? -more open policies for other health and social issues? -multi-sector and civil society engagement approaches adopted for other health issues? -capacity to plan and sustain health systems? |
| | | | | **What, if any, health improvements can be linked to PEPFAR's activities?** |
| *Human Resources* | What human resources have been introduced by PEPFAR? | What activities contributed to building capacity of workforce (pre-service, in-service)? What training programs exist for managers directed at - better service and planning: -performance assessment -CQI | What are the outputs of PEPFAR financed capacity building (number of people trained, by type of worker or training, in relation to the number of public workers, pre-service versus in-service): -percentage of HIV HCW paid vs. volunteer -percentage of PEPFAR trained workers transferred to/integrated with public sector  What are the outputs of PEFAR investments in HR, such as: -absolute number of new HCW added to the pool. -net number of new HCW added to pool (incoming versus lost workers) | To what extent are PEPFAR-financed capacity building activities supporting national HR plans for a sufficiently skilled HIV and non-HIV care workforce?  What are the outcomes of PEFAR investments in HR, such as: -retention of PEPFAR trained workers in public sectors versus non-governmental organizations, and in-country -urban-rural distribution HCW |

NOTE: CD4 = cluster of differentiation 4, CQI = continuous quality improvement, ELISA = enzyme-linked immunoabsorbent assay, HCW = health care worker, HHS = health systems strengthening, HR = human resources, QA = quality assessment, WHO = World Health Organization.